Transplant

Guest Editor

Darlene Lovasik, RN, MN, CCRN, CNRN

CRITICAL CARE NURSING CLINICS OF NORTH AMERICA

www.ccnursing.theclinics.com

Consulting Editor
JANET FOSTER, PhD, RN, CNS

September 2011 • Volume 23 • Number 3

SAUNDERS an imprint of ELSEVIER, Inc.

W.B. SAUNDERS COMPANY
A Division of Elsevier Inc.

Elsevier Inc., 1600 John F. Kennedy Blvd., Suite 1800, Philadelphia, PA 19103-2899

http://www.theclinics.com

CRITICAL CARE NURSING CLINICS OF NORTH AMERICA Volume 23, Number 3
September 2011 ISSN 0899-5885, ISBN-13: 978-1-4377-2439-4

Editor: Katie Hartner
Developmental Editor: Donald E. Mumford

Critical Care Nursing Clinics of North America (ISSN 0899-5885) is published quarterly by Elsevier Inc., 360 Park Avenue South, New York, NY 10010-1710. Months of issue are March, June, September, and December. Business and Editorial Offices: 1600 John F. Kennedy Blvd., Suite 1800, Philadelphia, PA 19103-2899. Periodicals postage paid at New York, NY and additional mailing offices. Subscription prices are $135.00 per year for US individuals, $282.00 per year for US institutions, $71.00 per year for US students and residents, $180.00 per year for Canadian individuals, $353.00 per year for Canadian institutions, $206.00 per year for international individuals, $353.00 per year for international institutions and $104.00 per year for Canadian and foreign students/residents. To receive student/resident rate, orders must be accompanied by name of affiliated institution, data of term, and the *signature* of program/residency coordinator on institution letterhead. Orders will be billed at individual rate until proof of status is received. Foreign air speed delivery is included in all *Clinics* subscription prices. All prices are subject to change without notice. **POSTMASTER:** Send address changes to *Critical Care Nursing Clinics of North America*, Elsevier Health Sciences Division, Subscription Customer Service, 3251 Riverport Lane, Maryland Heights, MO 63043. **Customer Service: 1-800-654-2452 (US and Canada); 314-447-8871 (outside US and Canada). Fax: 314-447-8029. E-mail: JournalsCustomerService-usa@elsevier.com (for print support) and JournalsOnlineSupport-usa@elsevier.com (for online support).**

Reprints. For copies of 100 or more of articles in this publication, please contact the Commercial Reprints Department, Elsevier Inc., 360 Park Avenue South, New York, New York, 10010-1710; Tel.: (212) 633-3813, Fax: (212) 462-1935, and E-mail: reprints@elsevier.com.

Critical Care Nursing Clinics of North America is covered in *MEDLINE/PubMed (Index Medicus), International Nursing Index, Nursing Citation Index, Cumulative Index to Nursing and Allied Health Literature,* and *RNdex Top 100.*

Printed and bound by CPI Group (UK) Ltd, Croydon, CR0 4YY

Transferred to Digital Print 2011

Contributors

CONSULTING EDITOR

JANET FOSTER, PhD, CNS
Texas Woman's University, College of Nursing, Houston, Texas

GUEST EDITOR

DARLENE LOVASIK, RN, MN, CCRN, CNRN
UPMC Presbyterian, Pittsburgh, Pennsylvania

AUTHORS

JENNIFER BOWMAN, RN, BSN, MBA
Transplant Coordinator, Cardiothoracic Transplant Institute, UPMC Presbyterian, University of Pittsburgh Medical Center, Pittsburgh, Pennsylvania

GERALD BRANDACHER, MD
Department of Plastic and Reconstructive Surgery, Johns Hopkins University School of Medicine, Baltimore, MD

SANDRA A. CUPPLES, PhD, RN
Washington Hospital Center, Washington, DC

JEANNINE V. DINELLA, RN, MSN
Advanced Practice Nurse Cardiology, Department of Nursing, UPMC Presbyterian, University of Pittsburgh Medical Center, Pittsburgh, Pennsylvania

DANIEL E. FOUST, RN, BSN
UPMC Presbyterian, Pittsburgh, Pennsylvania

ELISABETH L. GEORGE, RN, PhD
Advanced Practice Nurse Critical Care, Department of Nursing, University of Pittsburgh Medical Center–Presbyterian Shadyside, Pittsburgh, Pennsylvania

VIJAY S. GORANTLA, MD, PhD
Division of Plastic and Reconstructive Surgery, University of Pittsburgh School of Medicine, Pittsburgh, PA

TRACY A. GROGAN, RN, MEd, BSN, CCRN, CCTN
Unit Director, Transplant Intensive Care Unit, University of Pittsburgh Medical Center, Presbyterian-Shadyside, Pittsburgh, Pennsylvania

JANE GUTTENDORF, RN, MSN, CRNP, ACNP-BC
Acute Care Nurse Practitioner, Cardiothoracic ICU, Department of Critical Care Medicine, University of Pittsburgh Medical Center–Presbyterian Shadyside, Pittsburgh, Pennsylvania

MICHELLE M. JAMES, MS, RN, CNS, CCTN
Solid Organ Transplant Clinical Nurse Specialist, Department of Nursing, University of Minnesota Medical Center, Fairview, Minneapolis, Minnesota

W.P. ANDREW LEE, MD
Department of Plastic and Reconstructive Surgery, Johns Hopkins University School of Medicine, Baltimore, MD

JOSEPH E. LOSEE, MD
Division of Plastic and Reconstructive Surgery, University of Pittsburgh School of Medicine, Pittsburgh, PA

DARLENE LOVASIK, RN, MN, CCRN, CNRN
UPMC Presbyterian, Pittsburgh, Pennsylvania

DEANNA MCCAFFERY, RN, MSN, CCTN
Senior Professional Staff Nurse, Abdominal Transplant ICU, University of Pittsburgh Medical Center, Pittsburgh, Pennsylvania

MARY SHEELA PALOCAREN, RN, MSN, CCTN
Primary Nurse Care Coordinator, Abdominal Transplantation, UPMC Presbyterian, University of Pittsburgh Medical Center, Pittsburgh, Pennsylvania

KRISTINE S. SCHONDER, PharmD
Assistant Professor, Department of Pharmacy and Therapeutics University of Pittsburgh School of Pharmacy; Clinical Pharmacist, Ambulatory Care and Transplantation, Thomas E. Starzl Transplantation Institute, Pittsburgh, Pennsylvania

Contents

Transplantation has been an accepted treatment for end-stage organ disease for more than 30 years. Advances in transplant immunology are the cornerstone to the success of the body's ability to accept the allografted organ while continuing to perform immune functions such as tumor surveillance and fighting pathogenic organisms. This article describes immunosuppressant regimens and attendant nursing considerations in the care of transplant patients.

Substantial progress has been made in the past 3 decades in solid organ transplantation. The discovery of potent immunosuppressive agents capable of sustaining graft function with relatively minimal toxicity has paved the way to allow more patients to receive not only a solid organ transplant, but also more types of organs, and now even tissues, to be transplanted. As a result, solid organ transplant is a viable treatment option for many types of end-organ disease, including chronic kidney disease, liver failure, chronic heart failure, type I diabetes mellitus, chronic lung disease, and diseases that affect the small bowel.

Pancreas transplantation has been successful for restoring euglycemia in persons with type 1 diabetes mellitus. The transplantation may be performed as a single procedure, or it may follow or be performed simultaneous with kidney transplantation. This article discusses potential consequences of hyperglycemia and hypoglycemia and indications, alternatives, and contraindications for transplantation. The author also describes postoperative nursing care and potential complications including surgical and immunologic. Potential outcomes of pancreas transplantation can include survival benefit, physiologic improvement, and enhanced quality of life.

Liver transplantation has evolved into an accepted treatment for many suffering from end-stage liver failure. The clinical care and condition of the patient before transplant can impact the outcome after transplant. This article describes postoperative assessments of the patient's status and the integral role nurses can play in early identification of graft dysfunction, rejection, or infection. The nurse is often in a position to monitor for potential risks to the patient and take corrective action.

Intestine transplantation remains a formidable clinical and immunologic challenge. With newer immunosuppression and accumulated experience, survival outcomes are improving. The relationship of recipient preexisting conditions with the risk of postoperative events emphasizes the necessity of early referral to expert transplant programs before the onset of life-threatening complications. Improved patient outcomes after intestine and multivisceral transplant will be achieved with increased awareness and knowledge regarding referral criteria, transplant criteria, optimal time for transplantation, and medication regimens.

Today, heart transplantation is a viable treatment option for end-stage disease for patients at almost any age. This article discusses the current information related to caring for heart transplant patients. Topics covered include pathophysiology, workup, waiting list, preparation, procedure, rejection, infection, complications, and nursing care.

The modern era of transplantation began in the 1980s with the introduction of cyclosporine. Current volume statistics indicate that lung transplantation is a recognized option for select patients with end-stage lung disease. Based on Organ Procurement and Transplant Network data as of April 16, 2010, 19,907 patients have undergone isolated lung transplant and 1027 patients have undergone heart-lung procedures. Because of advancements in immunosuppression, surgical techniques, donor selection and criteria, and preoperative and postoperative patient management, there have been marked improvement in outcomes since the 1990s.

Preface

Transplantation: Past, Present, and Future

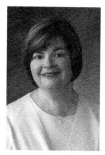

Darlene Lovasik, RN, MN, CCRN, CNRN
Guest Editor

A kidney was transplanted from one healthy identical twin to his twin who was dying of renal disease on December 23, 1954. The operation was successful; renal function was restored in the recipient, and the donor remained in good health. This pioneering surgery kept the recipient alive for eight years; the donor lived a healthy life and died at age 79 in 2010, and lead surgeon Dr Joseph Murray went on to win the Nobel Prize. The early drugs used to treat rejection for kidney transplant, azathioprine and corticosteroids, were also used in the initial efforts at liver, heart, and pancreas surgery, but patient mortality was high. In the early 1980s, cyclosporin, a calcineurin inhibitor, was introduced and led to a striking reduction in rejection for kidney transplants as well as marked improvement in outcomes for liver and heart transplant recipients. Other immunosuppressive drugs, tacrolimus, mycophenolate mofetil, and sirolimus (with different profiles and efficacy), were introduced in the 1990s. To a great extent, transplantation advanced through the work of Thomas E. Starzl, MD, PhD, whose foresight, perseverance, and commitment made him the modern-day father of organ transplantation, and none of these triumphs would have been achieved if our transplant leaders had not first undertaken exacting laboratory work to show that these operations would be feasible and effective. The success and progress in transplantation are also irrevocably linked to the developments in immunosuppressive therapy and immunomodulation strategies.

These advancements in the field of transplantation have given hope to thousands of patients facing organ failure. Since January 1, 1988, over 518,000 organ transplants have been performed in the United States. More than 406,000 organ-transplant recipients received organs from deceased donors, and over 112,000 recipients received organs, usually kidneys, from living donors. The medical specialists and surgeons who guide people to new lives as organ recipients, the nurses, clinical coordinators, and physicians who provide care and support before and after surgery, and the researchers who move

Crit Care Nurs Clin N Am 23 (2011) ix–x
doi:10.1016/j.ccell.2011.09.003
0899-5885/11/$ – see front matter © 2011 Elsevier Inc. All rights reserved.

the field forward have continued to innovate and lead efforts to discover new and better therapies to help reduce the potential for organ rejection.

This issue of *Critical Care Nursing Clinics of North America* is a collection of articles on transplantation. The authors provided vital information for organ-specific assessment and nursing interventions for recipients of pancreas, liver, intestine/multivisceral, heart, lung, and upper extremity transplant, discussed aspects of care that are common in all transplant recipients, including organ rejection, risk of infection, and physical and psychosocial problems, and reviewed immunosuppressive drug therapy and, the potential complications.

As graft and patient survival improves, it is no longer necessary for these patients to return to their transplant center for hospital admissions that are not related to their transplanted organ; however, the patient's transplant status must be a significant part of the plan of care. Transplant recipients will develop the same health problems as other aging individuals; however, they are likely to develop these conditions earlier and their diseases will progress at an accelerated rate. Optimal patient care is achieved through close collaboration between community health care providers and the transplant centers.

As the guest editor of this issue of *Critical Care Nursing Clinics of North America*, I would like to thank each of the contributing authors for sharing their time, energy, and clinical expertise on caring for the transplant patients with their professional colleagues. I am grateful for the supportive relationships that I have with the physicians, nurses, pharmacists, and other health care professionals who work with this challenging patient population and hope that you also have the benefit of true collaboration in your work environment. For her patience and support, I would also like to thank Katie Hartner from Elsevier. And a final "thank you" to the patients and families, whose courage, grace, and dignity continue to inspire us.

Darlene Lovasik, RN, MN, CCRN, CNRN
UPMC Presbyterian
N1274, Unit 12 North, MUH
200 Lothrop Street
Pittsburgh, PA 15213, USA

E-mail address:
lovasikdj@upmc.edu

A Review of Transplant Immunology

Deanna McCaffery, RN, MSN, CCTN

KEYWORDS
- Transplant immunology • Allografted organs
- Immunosuppression • Nursing considerations

Transplantation has been an accepted treatment for end-stage organ disease for more than 30 years. Advances in transplant immunology are the cornerstone to the success of the body's ability to accept the allografted organ while continuing to perform immune functions such as tumor surveillance and fighting pathogenic organisms. The history of transplant immunology has been written through the work of physicians such as Medewar, Gorer, Murray, and Starzl. Modifying the immune response to promote tolerance and chimerism through pharmacology has greatly extended the survival rates of liver transplant recipients. Current trends in immunosuppression focus on both allograft function and the recipient's quality of life.

Following the determined efforts of transplant pioneers, transplantation is now considered a viable therapeutic modality for kidney, pancreas, liver, intestine, heart, and lung end-stage organ disease as well as composite tissue allotransplantation (face, hands, larynx, muscle flaps, and others). Success in the field of transplantation was built on the scientific advances in immunology. Suppressing the immune system's ability to recognize self from nonself is the key to survival of the transplanted organ and, ultimately, the patient. Advances in transplant immunology have led to short-term survival rates being replaced with long-term survival rates as clinical indicators of success. Immunosuppressive regimens that prevent rejection and prolong allograft survival often carry serious side effects to both the allografted organ and the recipient. Greater understanding of the immune response has shifted the focus of transplant immunology to tolerance and chimerism, concepts that are key to long-term allograft survival and the recipient's quality of life.[1]

THE IMMUNE RESPONSE

In animals, lymphocytes are the cells responsible for the immune response and can be divided into five groups. These groups are based on function and specific surface

Transplant ICU, UPMC Presbyterian, University of Pittsburgh Medical Center, 200 Lothrop Street, Pittsburgh, PA 15213, USA
* Corresponding author.
E-mail address: deannamccaffery@gmail.com

Crit Care Nurs Clin N Am 23 (2011) 393–404
doi:10.1016/j.ccell.2011.08.004
0899-5885/11/$ – see front matter © 2011 Elsevier Inc. All rights reserved.

compounds: B lymphocytes, accessory cells (macrophages), natural killer cells (NK and NKT cells), and mast cells. Each of these groups performs specific functions correlated to the surface receptors that they possess. When the appropriate antigen is encountered, the lymphocyte produces immunoglobulins (antigen-specific antibodies), proliferates, and differentiates. Because the lymphocyte's reaction is greater the second time it encounters the antigen, it demonstrates that immune responses are specific and acquire memory. This function is an integral theory in transplant immunology.

B cells and macrophages break down proteins, including bacteria, and display antigens (short peptide chains) on the cell's surface through the major histocompatibility complex (MHC). Both normal proteins (self) and microbial pathogens (nonself) are present (**Fig. 1**). The MHC signals the immune system that nonself or foreign substance is there. The T cells or NK cells survey the surface and if a MHC peptide is recognized, it activates the immune cell, producing an immune response. Helper T cells then stimulate B cells to develop antibodies. B cells divide and differentiate to form antibody-secreting plasma cells that bind to bacteria so that they can be ingested by macrophages. This is the key to producing monoclonal antibodies.

Antibodies recognize antigens in their native state (humoral immunity), but T cells recognize only antigens in fragmented forms (cell-mediated immunity). When an antibody recognizes an antigen, it triggers a host of cell-mediated clearing processes (phagocytosis) against the live microorganisms. Peptide fragments derived from intercellular protein synthesis are displayed on the cell surface bound to MHC 1 molecules. Phagocyte extracellular proteins are bound to the cell surface by MHC 2 molecules.

T cells are integral to the cell-mediated responses of the immune system. Interfering with the cell's ability to recognize the allograft as an antigen is the primary way that rejection is avoided. Since the development of cyclosporine (and later immunosuppressive agents), transplant pharmacology has concentrated its efforts on T-cell alteration.

MODIFYING THE IMMUNE RESPONSE

Down-regulation of the immune system is crucial to the survival of the allografted organ. Because the allograft is not self-limiting, immunosuppressant must be maintained throughout the patient's life. Two strategies are used to achieve down-regulation: immunotherapy and tolerance induction. Numerous immunosuppressive therapies have been developed over the last 50 years; however, the concept of immune tolerance or immunologic tolerance that is currently studied in the transplant community is either immunosuppressive-free or minimal dosage. Three things are considered when designing the immunosuppressant regimen: the immunosuppressive load must be low enough for T cells to respond to infective organisms and to carry out tumor surveillance, decreasing tumor surveillance increases the risk of malignancy and can result in posttransplant lymphoproliferative disease (PTLD), and damage to the allograft must be circumvented by the allergenic response. Complementary agents should also be used to optimize the efficacy of the immunosuppressant and decrease its toxicity to the recipient.[2]

Long-term survival is now the clinical indicator for success in transplantation. Quality of life is as important a goal as a well functioning allograft for transplant recipients to live a normal life span. Because the immunosuppressant agents have many side effects, the quality of life greatly improves if the transplant recipient's

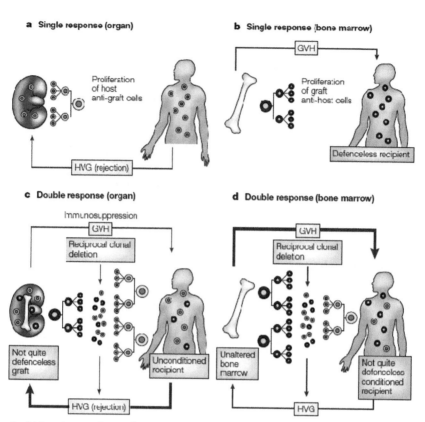

a Single response (organ)

Proliferation of host anti-graft cells

HVG (rejection)

b Single response (bone marrow)

GVH

Proliferation of graft anti-host cells

Defenceless recipient

c Double response (organ)

Immunosuppression

GVH

Reciprocal clonal deletion

Not quite defenceless graft

Unconditioned recipient

HVG (rejection)

d Double response (bone marrow)

GVH

Reciprocal clonal deletion

Unaltered bone marrow

Not quite defenceless conditioned recipient

HVG

Fig. 1. Old and new views of transplantation immunology. (*a*) Early conceptualization of immune mechanisms in organ transplantation in terms of a unidirectional host-versus-graft (HVG) response. (*b*) A mirror image of (*a*) depicting the early understanding of successful bone marrow (BM) transplantation as a complete replacement of the recipient immune system by that of the donor, with the potential complication of an unopposed lethal unidirectional graft-versus-host (GVH) response, ie, rejection of the recipient by the graft. (*c*) Current view of bidirectional and reciprocally modulating immune responses of coexisting immunocompetent cell populations that lead to organ engraftment, despite a usually dominant HVG reaction. The transplanted organ, which initially loses most of its passenger leukocytes, apparently remains an important site for donor precursor and stem cells (bone silhouette). (*d*) The current conceived mirror image of (*c*) showing the reversal of the size proportions of the reciprocally modulating donor and recipient populations of immune cells after successful BM transplantation. (*From* Starzl TE, Zinkernagel RM. Transplantation tolerance from a historical perspective. Nat Rev Immunology 2001;1:239; with permission.

immune system can be trained to tolerate the allografted organ without immunosuppressive medications. Tolerance is a state of antigen-specific T-cell unresponsiveness with minimal immunosuppressant. The T cell responds to all other antigens, but has no or minimal response to a specific antigen connected with the allografted organ. Induction agents are used as conditioning immediately before transplantation or given during transplant surgery to promote tolerance in long-term liver transplant recipients. There are two primary agents: alemtuzumab (Campath) is a monoclonal antibody that rapidly purges T and B lymphocytes, and thymoglobulin (RATG is used for transplant) targets and damages T lymphocytes only. Both agents alter the immune response and increase the risk of infection; however, alemtuzumab reduces B lymphocytes for several months and T lymphocytes for up to 1 to 3 years, reducing the risk of rejection, although it increases the risk of infection.

A "chimera" is an organism composed of two or more genetically distinct cells. In transplantation, chimerism indicates the coexistence of donor and recipient cells; the donor hemopoietic cells survive with recipient hemopoietic cells. With immunosuppressants, the donor cells endure and the recipient's blood is populated with both donor human leukocyte antigen (HLA) type and recipient HLA type. Because "self" now includes both donor and recipient cells, the immune response is diminished.[2] Some recipients have survived more than 25 years with their transplanted organs, which suggests that chimerism after organ transplantation may be a naturally occurring event. Other recipients may have functioning organs while on little or no immunosuppressive drugs, indicating that a functional donor-specific tolerance has occurred. This continues to be an exciting area of investigation for transplant researchers in basic science and clinical studies.

TRANSPLANT IMMUOLOGY

Medawar is credited with being the father of transplant immunology. He documented the presence of "graft-versus-host" disease in 1944. During the 1940s, he used total body irradiation on rats undergoing skin grafts. Total body radiation failed when it was applied to humans; rejection was not prevented and lethal infections resulted.[3]

Surgical techniques for kidney and liver transplantation were perfected in the canine laboratory by various physicians during the 1950s and early 1960s. Without the ability to suppress the immune system, all of these transplant recipients died of allograft rejection. In 1968, azathioprine (Imuran) was approved by the FDA for use in organ transplantation; azathioprine inhibits DNA replication of lymphocytes. Murray performed the first successful kidney transplant on identical twins, but was unable to prevent rejection in kidney transplants using azathioprine alone. Starzl combined azathioprine with corticosteroids to establish the immunosuppressive regimen that was used for all solid organ transplants for the next 20 years. Polyclonal antibody production began in the late 1960s as a result of using horse and rabbit serum immunized with human lymphocytes or thymocytes to produce specific antibodies against T-cell receptors. Starzl introduced the anti-lymphoid globulin thymoglobulin as an induction agent before the first successful liver transplant in 1967.[3]

The MHC was first discovered by Gorer, Lymen, and Snell in 1970.[4] The MHC contains the genetic locus that encodes antigens associated with allograft rejection, tumor surveillance, and other cell-mediated responses. Cytotoxic lymphocytes recognize host cells as nonself through the MHC–peptide complexes displayed by the allograft. The detection of MHC led to the detection of human leukocyte antigen (HLA) proteins and the resultant tissue matching of the donor and recipient. Negative cross-matching of donor and recipient is necessary to avoid antibody-mediated rejection; a positive crossmatch signifies that the recipient's cells would attack the donor's cells and damage the donor's implanted organ. At this time, kidneys are the only transplant organs that are prospectively HLA-matched.

Although polyclonal antibodies were successful as induction agents owing to their ability to suppress T-cell production, monoclonal antibody development provided transplant immunology with powerful weapons against acute, steroid-resistant allograft rejection.

The discovery of the first calcineurin inhibitor, cyclosporine, altered the practice of organ transplantation by dramatically increasing allograft survival rates. Cyclosporine blocks interleukin-2 (IL-2) transcription on the T cell by binding to the protein cyclophilin that then inhibits lymphokine production. Another milestone in transplant immunology was reached in 1989 when recipient leukocytes were found in the bone marrow of successful bone marrow transplant recipients. Donor lymphocytes existing side by side with recipient lymphocytes led to the realization that chimerism exists in successful long-term transplantation. In 1989, the Japanese laboratory Fujisawa developed the calcineurin inhibitor FK506, now known as tacrolimus. Tacrolimus inhibits IL-2 synthesis by binding to the T cell's FK506 protein and blocking lymphokine transcription.[4] Transplant survival rates increased after Starzl pioneered use of FK506 for transplant recipients at the University of Pittsburgh. The side effects of tacrolimus are similar to, but less severe, than those of cyclosporine. The side effects of the calcineurin inhibitors include nephrotoxicity, liver toxicity, hypertension (decreased with tacrolimus), neurotoxicity, and diabetes (increased with tacrolimus). Calcineurin inhibitors continue to be the cornerstone of immunosuppressive regimens at transplant centers worldwide.

NURSING CONSIDERATIONS

Understanding the immune system's response to the allograft and the pharmacology of immunosuppressive medications, and recognizing the adverse effects of the immunosuppressant agents are vital to providing patient-focused bedside care. Patient quality of life is at the core of the nursing profession, and improving quality of life is one of the latest outcome measures in transplantation. Familiarity with the signs of infection, rejection, the complexity of the pharmacologic regimen, and sharing this information with the patient and caregivers is essential in providing exceptional nursing care for the transplant patient population. The goal of the entire transplant team is graft and patient survival while maintaining long-term quality of life.

CURRENT TRENDS

The story of transplant immunology is unfinished. Because the immune responses of the allograft and the recipient are the primary barriers to success in transplantation medicine, new approaches to inducing immunologic tolerance and chimerism are integrated into clinical trials. Pharmacologic immunosuppression has increased allograft survival rates dramatically over the last 20 years. The 1-year, 3-year, and 5-year graft and patient survival rates for organ transplantation have increased remarkably (**Tables 1** and **2**).[5] Immunosuppression increases risk of both cancer and infection and long-term use may lead to allograft damage and chronic rejection. These common complications of transplantation will be eliminated if tolerance can be achieved in the absence of pharmacologic immunosuppressants. Tolerance can be grouped into two categories: central (occurs in the thymus) and peripheral (occurs in the mature lymphocyte compartments). Both central and peripheral tolerances have advantages and concerns.[4] Transplant researchers have explored the use of bone marrow augmentation, white blood cell (WBC) transfusions, and induction therapy to induce tolerance. The option of steroid-free immunosuppressive therapy in the era of calcineurin inhibitors has decreased patient morbidity and chronic organ rejection and resulted in longer allograft survival.[6]

Results from recent and current clinical trials indicate that advances in tolerance induction will come from a combination of pharmacology, biological agents, and gene therapy.[7] As transplant immunology moves forward, the challenges of achieving tolerance and chimerism will be in the forefront of transplant research.

Table 1
Graft survival rates

Region	Organ	Recipient Gender	Years Posttransplant	Number Functioning/Alive	Survival Rate	95% Confidence Interval
U.S.	Heart–Lung	Male	1 Year	25	55.6	(40.3, 70.8)
U.S.	Heart–Lung	Female	1 Year	41	71.9	(59.0, 84.9)
U.S.	Heart–Lung	Male	3 Year	27	44.3	(31.6, 56.9)
U.S.	Heart–Lung	Female	3 Year	48	50.8	(40.6, 61.0)
U.S.	Heart–Lung	Male	5 Year	29	35.2	(25.0, 45.3)
U.S.	Heart–Lung	Female	5 Year	45	39.4	(30.6, 48.1)
U.S.	Heart	Male	1 Year	3933	87.5	(86.5, 88.4)
U.S.	Heart	Female	1 Year	1433	85.6	(83.8, 87.3)
U.S.	Heart	Male	3 Year	4860	78.9	(77.8, 79.9)
U.S.	Heart	Female	3 Year	1730	76.0	(74.2, 77.8)
U.S.	Heart	Male	5 Year	4518	72.4	(71.3, 73.5)
U.S.	Heart	Female	5 Year	1494	67.4	(65.5, 69.4)
U.S.	Intestine	Male	1 Year	148	80.2	(74.0, 86.4)
U.S.	Intestine	Female	1 Year	136	73.6	(66.8, 80.3)
U.S.	Intestine	Male	3 Year	87	47.5	(40.3, 54.7)
U.S.	Intestine	Female	3 Year	99	55.3	(47.8, 62.8)
U.S.	Intestine	Male	5 Year	62	39.1	(31.6, 46.7)
U.S.	Intestine	Female	5 Year	49	40.1	(31.5, 48.6)
U.S.	Kidney	Male	1 Year	24,346	91.4	(91.1, 91.8)
U.S.	Kidney	Female	1 Year	16,580	91.8	(91.4, 92.2)
U.S.	Kidney	Male	3 Year	24,459	81.9	(81.5, 82.3)
U.S.	Kidney	Female	3 Year	16,931	81.8	(81.3, 82.3)

(continued on next page)

Table 1
(continued)

Region	Organ	Recipient Gender	Years Posttransplant	Number Functioning/Alive	Survival Rate	95% Confidence Interval
U.S.	Kidney	Male	5 Year	17,931	71.2	(70.6, 71.7)
U.S.	Kidney	Female	5 Year	12,583	71.6	(71.0, 72.2)
U.S.	Kidney–pancreas	Male	1 Year	1463	91.7	(90.3, 93.1)
U.S.	Kidney–pancreas	Female	1 Year	930	91.6	(89.8, 93.4)
U.S.	Kidney–pancreas	Male	3 Year	1732	84.8	(83.2, 86.3)
U.S.	Kidney–pancreas	Female	3 Year	1142	82.7	(80.6, 84.7)
U.S.	Kidney–pancreas	Male	5 Year	1479	77.6	(75.8, 79.5)
U.S.	Kidney–pancreas	Female	5 Year	1003	73.9	(71.6, 76.2)
U.S.	Liver	Male	1 Year	9010	82.2	(81.5, 82.9)
U.S.	Liver	Female	1 Year	4884	81.8	(80.8, 82.8)
U.S.	Liver	Male	3 Year	8654	72.1	(71.3, 72.9)
U.S.	Liver	Female	3 Year	5254	71.8	(70.8, 72.8)
U.S.	Liver	Male	5 Year	6483	64.9	(64.0, 65.8)
U.S.	Liver	Female	5 Year	4453	65.4	(64.3, 66.5)
U.S.	Lung	Male	1 Year	1379	82.5	(80.6, 84.3)
U.S.	Lung	Female	1 Year	1324	82.6	(80.7, 84.5)
U.S.	Lung	Male	3 Year	1159	61.0	(58.8, 63.2)
U.S.	Lung	Female	3 Year	1241	62.3	(60.2, 64.5)
U.S.	Lung	Male	5 Year	802	45.4	(43.1, 47.8)
U.S.	Lung	Female	5 Year	814	46.1	(43.8, 48.4)
U.S.	Pancreas	Male	1 Year	673	78.8	(76.0, 81.6)
U.S.	Pancreas	Female	1 Year	564	74.9	(71.7, 78.1)

(continued on next page)

Table 1
(continued)

Region	Organ	Recipient Gender	Years Posttransplant	Number Functioning/Alive	Survival Rate	95% Confidence Interval
U.S.	Pancreas	Male	3 Year	573	66.3	(63.2, 69.4)
U.S.	Pancreas	Female	3 Year	489	62.3	(58.9, 65.7)
U.S.	Pancreas	Male	5 Year	298	54.1	(50.1, 58.0)
U.S.	Pancreas	Female	5 Year	242	48.7	(44.5, 52.9)

Data subject to change based on future data submission or correction.

[a]A graft survival was not computed due to N < 10. 1-year survival based on 2002–2004 transplants, 3-year survival based on 1999–2002 transplants, 5-year survival based on 1997–2000 transplants.

Data from Organ Procurement and Transplantation Network. All Kaplan–Meier graft survival rates for transplants performed: 1997–2004. OPTN data as of July 22, 2011. Available at: http://optn.transplant.hrsa.gov/latestData/rptStrat.asp. Accessed July 29, 2011.

Table 2

Patient survival rates

Region	Organ	Recipient Gender	Years Post Transplant	Number Functioning/Alive	Survival Rate	95% Confidence Interval
U.S.	Heart–lung	Male	1 Year	25	55.6	(40.3, 70.8)
U.S.	Heart–lung	Female	1 Year	41	74.8	(61.9, 87.7)
U.S.	Heart–lung	Male	3 Year	27	44.3	(31.6, 56.9)
U.S.	Heart–lung	Female	3 Year	48	53.4	(43.0, 63.9)
U.S.	Heart–lung	Male	5 Year	29	35.8	(25.5, 46.0)
U.S.	Heart–lung	Female	5 Year	45	41.4	(32.4, 50.5)
U.S.	Heart	Male	1 Year	3933	88.0	(87.0, 89.0)
U.S.	Heart	Female	1 Year	1433	86.2	(84.5, 87.9)
U.S.	Heart	Male	3 Year	4860	79.3	(78.3, 80.4)
U.S.	Heart	Female	3 Year	1730	77.2	(75.5, 79.0)
U.S.	Heart	Male	5 Year	4518	73.2	(72.1, 74.2)
U.S.	Heart	Female	5 Year	1494	69.0	(67.1, 70.9)
U.S.	Intestine	Male	1 Year	148	82.2	(76.2, 88.2)
U.S.	Intestine	Female	1 Year	136	75.0	(68.4, 81.7)
U.S.	Intestine	Male	3 Year	87	57.0	(49.4, 64.6)
U.S.	Intestine	Female	3 Year	99	60.1	(52.5, 67.7)
U.S.	Intestine	Male	5 Year	62	49.0	(40.6, 57.4)
U.S.	Intestine	Female	5 Year	49	45.5	(36.3, 54.6)
U.S.	Kidney	Male	1 Year	25,171	95.6	(95.4, 95.9)
U.S.	Kidney	Female	1 Year	17,198	96.3	(96.1, 96.6)
U.S.	Kidney	Male	3 Year	25,738	90.3	(89.9, 90.6)
U.S.	Kidney	Female	3 Year	17,928	91.3	(90.9, 91.7)
U.S.	Kidney	Male	5 Year	19,315	84.2	(83.8, 84.7)

(continued on next page)

Table 2
(continued)

Region	Organ	Recipient Gender	Years Post Transplant	Number Functioning/Alive	Survival Rate	95% Confidence Interval
U.S.	Kidney	Female	5 Year	13,578	85.8	(85.2, 86.3)
U.S.	Kidney/Pancreas	Male	1 Year	1484	94.4	(93.2, 95.6)
U.S.	Kidney/Pancreas	Female	1 Year	954	95.5	(94.1, 96.9)
U.S.	Kidney/Pancreas	Male	3 Year	1757	90.3	(89.0, 91.6)
U.S.	Kidney/Pancreas	Female	3 Year	1170	89.5	(87.8, 91.1)
U.S.	Kidney/Pancreas	Male	5 Year	1530	86.1	(84.5, 87.7)
U.S.	Kidney/Pancreas	Female	5 Year	1037	84.6	(82.6, 86.5)
U.S.	Liver	Male	1 Year	9010	86.7	(86.0, 87.3)
U.S.	Liver	Female	1 Year	4884	86.1	(85.2, 87.0)
U.S.	Liver	Male	3 Year	8654	78.3	(77.6, 79.1)
U.S.	Liver	Female	3 Year	5254	78.3	(77.3, 79.3)
U.S.	Liver	Male	5 Year	6483	71.8	(70.9, 72.7)
U.S.	Liver	Female	5 Year	4453	73.0	(71.9, 74.1)
U.S.	Lung	Male	1 Year	1379	83.2	(81.3, 85.0)
U.S.	Lung	Female	1 Year	1324	83.4	(81.6, 85.3)
U.S.	Lung	Male	3 Year	1159	62.2	(60.0, 64.4)
U.S.	Lung	Female	3 Year	1241	63.1	(61.0, 65.3)
U.S.	Lung	Male	5 Year	802	46.6	(44.3, 49.0)
U.S.	Lung	Female	5 Year	814	47.3	(44.9, 49.6)
U.S.	Pancreas	Male	1 Year	793	95.0	(93.4, 96.6)
U.S.	Pancreas	Female	1 Year	677	93.4	(91.4, 95.3)

(continued on next page)

Table 2
(continued)

Region	Organ	Recipient Gender	Years Post Transplant	Number Functioning/Alive	Survival Rate	95% Confidence Interval
U.S.	Pancreas	Male	3 Year	659	90.2	(88.1, 92.3)
U.S.	Pancreas	Female	3 Year	570	88.8	(86.5, 91.2)
U.S.	Pancreas	Male	5 Year	337	84.6	(81.4, 87.8)
U.S.	Pancreas	Female	5 Year	278	79.0	(75.1, 83.0)

Data subject to change based on future data submission or correction.

[a]A graft survival was not computed due to $N < 10$. 1-year survival based on 2002–2004 transplants, 3-year survival based on 1999–2002 transplants, 5-year survival based on 1997–2000 transplants.

Data from Organ Procurement and Transplantation Network. All Kaplan–Meier graft survival rates for transplants performed: 1997–2004. OPTN data as of July 22, 2011. Available at: http://optn.transplant.hrsa.gov/llatestData/rptStrat.asp. Accessed July 29, 2011.

In the words of Thomas E. Starzl, "The lesson is clear. History is neither dull nor dead. It is an uniquely human survival tool, aiding those in the present by the ability to draw on the past to meet current needs and to predict needs yet to come."[8]

REFERENCES

1. Starzl TE. Acquired immunologic tolerance: with particular reference to transplantation. Immunol Res 2007;38(1–3):6–41.
2. Starzl TE, Murase N, Abu-Elmagd K, et al. Tolerogenic immunosuppression for organ transplantation. Lancet 2000;361(9368):1502–10.
3. Starzl TE. The saga of liver replacement, with particular reference to the reciprocal influence of liver and kidney transplantation (1955–1967). J Am Coll Surg 2002;195(5): 587–610.
4. Smith SL. Historical perspective of transplantation. Organ Transplant 2002;1–8. Available at: http://www.medscape.com/viewarticle/436532. Accessed December 18, 2007.
5. Organ Procurement and Transplantation Network (OPTN). Available at: http://optn. transplant.hrsa.gov/latestData/rptStrat.asp. Accessed July 20, 2011.
6. Keown P. Improving quality of life—the new target for transplantation. Transplantation 2001;72(12 Suppl):S67–S74.
7. Heslan JM, Renaudin K, Thebault P, et al. New evidence for a role of allograft accommodation in long-term tolerance. Transplantation 2006;82(9):1185–93.
8. Starzl TE. The saga of liver replacement, with particular reference to the reciprocal influence of liver and kidney transplantation (1955–1967). J Am Coll Surg 2002;195(5): 587.

Pharmacology of Immunosuppressive Medications in Solid Organ Transplantation

Kristine S. Schonder, PharmD[a,b,*]

KEYWORDS

• Pharmacology • Immunosuppression
• Organ transplantation

THE CLINICAL AND ECONOMIC POTENTIAL OF CYCLOSPORINE DRUG INTERACTIONS

Substantial progress has been made in the past 3 decades in solid organ transplantation. The discovery of potent immunosuppressive agents capable of sustaining graft function with relatively minimal toxicity has paved the way to allow more patients to receive not only a solid organ transplant, but also more types of organs, and now even tissues, to be transplanted. As a result, solid organ transplant is a viable treatment option for many types of end-organ disease, including chronic kidney disease (CKD), liver failure, chronic heart failure, type I diabetes mellitus, chronic lung disease, and diseases that affect the small bowel.

Currently available immunosuppressive agents target T-lymphocyte activity, the primary mediator of rejection in solid organ transplantation. T-lymphocyte activity is greatest immediately after the transplant procedure when the T lymphocytes first become exposed to the foreign antigens. As a result, the degree of immunosuppression is greatest within the first months after transplantation. Immunosuppression in solid organ transplant becomes a delicate balance to maintain organ function and prevent acute rejection, while preventing the development of toxicity. The most common toxicity associated with all immunosuppressive medications is infectious complications. Thus, the risk of infections is also related to the degree of immunosuppression. As time lapses after the transplant, the risk of rejection decreases but is

[a] Department of Pharmacy and Therapeutics University of Pittsburgh School of Pharmacy, 200 Lothrop Street, PFG 01-01-01, Pittsburgh, PA 15213, USA
[b] Ambulatory Care and Transplantation, Thomas E. Starzl Transplantation Institute, Pittsburgh, PA, USA
* Corresponding author.
E-mail address: schonderks@upmc.edu

Crit Care Nurs Clin N Am 23 (2011) 405–423
doi:10.1016/j.ccell.2011.06.001
0899-5885/11/$ – see front matter © 2011 Elsevier Inc. All rights reserved.

not eliminated completely. Therefore, the degree, and thus drug doses, of immuno-suppression decreases but cannot be discontinued completely.

There are several strategies for managing immunosuppression after solid organ transplant. In general, all protocols involve combining several immunosuppressing agents that target different areas of T-lymphocyte activity to render the cells ineffective to mount a response to the foreign antigen. Many protocols will include induction therapy in an attempt to further suppress the immune system at the time of transplant, when the risk of rejection is greatest. Induction therapy involves admin-istering a potent immunosuppressant, usually an antibody that targets specific markers on the T lymphocyte, to block T-lymphocyte recognition or activity against the foreign antigens. Patients then receive maintenance immunosuppression, gener-ally a combination of drugs, for the life of the transplanted organ. In the event of an acute rejection episode, more potent immunosuppression is administered to stop the T-lymphocyte attack. High doses of steroids block T-lymphocyte recognition and decrease infiltration at the transplanted graft, whereas lymphocytic antibodies de-stroy activated T lymphocytes to reverse the rejection process.

The following discussion will describe the mechanism of action and relevant pharmacologic aspects associated with the immunosuppressants used in solid organ transplantation. Because maintenance immunosuppression is continued for the life of the transplanted organ, these drugs will be discussed first, followed by the antibody preparations that are used for induction therapy and treatment of rejection.

CALCINEURIN INHIBITORS

Calcineurin inhibitors are the foundation of most immunosuppressive regimens in solid organ transplantation. There are 2 calcineurin inhibitors currently available: cyclosporine and tacrolimus. The introduction of cyclosporine in the early 1980s brought with it a significant reduction in acute cellular rejection and severe infections, thereby dramatically improving graft and patient survival.[1] Today, tacrolimus is the most widely used calcineurin inhibitor for all solid organ transplants.[2]

Cyclosporine

Cyclosporine exerts its immunosuppressive effects by binding to cyclophilin, a cytoplasmic immunophilin. The resulting cyclosporine-cyclophilin complex inhibits the activity of calcineurin, a phosphatase responsible for activating the nuclear factor of activated T lymphocytes (NF-AT). NF-AT is the primary trigger responsible for initiating the transcription of cytokines responsible for the activity of T lymphocytes. One such cytokine is interleukin (IL)-2, which acts as a potent growth factor that promotes activation and proliferation of T lymphocytes.

There are 2 forms of cyclosporine currently available in the United States: cyclosporine, USP (Sandimmune®) and cyclosporine, USP [MODIFIED] (Neoral®). Cyclosporine, USP exhibits highly variable absorption because it is dependent on bile for absorption from the gastrointestinal (GI) tract. Absorption can range from 5% to 60%, and peak concentrations are reached within 2 to 6 hours. The variations in absorption are seen between patients and also within a single patient with consecutive doses. These fluctuations lead to difficulty with dosing and maintaining adequate levels to prevent acute rejection. The microemulsion formulation of cyclosporine, USP [MOD-IFIED] allows the product to emulsify readily in the GI fluids, which makes the product less dependent on bile for absorption and more easily absorbed. The result is a more predictable absorption of 60% with peak concentrations being reached within 1.5 to 2 hours. Cyclosporine absorption is decreased in African American patients com-pared with Caucasians, regardless of the formulation.[3]

Table 1
Adverse reactions associated with maintenance immunosuppressants

	CSA	TAC	Steroids	MMF	AZA	SIR	EVL
Alopecia		X			X		
Anemia				X[a]	X[a]	X	X
Diarrhea, nausea		X		X	X	X	X
GI bleeding			X				
Gingival hyperplasia	X						
Hirsutism	X						
Hyperglycemia	X	X	X				
Hyperkalemia, hypomagnesemia	X	X					
Hyperlipidemia	X	X	X			X	X
Hypertension	X	X	X				
Hyperuricemia	X	X					
Insomnia	X	X	X				
Leukocytosis			X				
Leukopenia				X[a]	X[a]	X[a]	X[a]
Mood changes			X				
Nephrotoxicity	X[a]	X[a]				X	X
Neurotoxicity (tremors, headache)	X[a]	X[a]					
Thrombocytopenia				X[a]	X[a]	X	X
Weight gain			X				
Proteinuria						X	X

Abbreviations: AZA, Azathioprine; CSA, cyclosporine; EVL, everolimus; MMF, mycophenolate mofetil; SIR, sirolimus; TAC, tacrolimus.
[a] Indicates dose-limiting adverse effect.

Once absorbed, 90% of cyclosporine is bound to plasma lipoproteins and widely distributed into tissues and body fluids. The volume of distribution can range from 3 to 5 L/kg. Cyclosporine is metabolized in the liver by cytochrome P450 (CYP) 3A4 enzymes and acts as a substrate for p-glycoprotein (PGP) in the GI tract and the liver. Similar to the differences in absorption, elimination half-life also differs between the 2 cyclosporine products. Cyclosporine, USP has an average half-life of 19 hours, but can range from 10 to 27 hours because of enterohepatic recycling of the drug via bile. Cyclosporine, USP [MODIFIED], however, has a more predictable half-life that averages 8 hours and ranges from 5 to 18 hours.

Adverse effects of cyclosporine include both metabolic and cosmetic effects (see **Table 1**). The dose-limiting toxicities of cyclosporine are nephrotoxicity and neurotoxicity. Nephrotoxicity is caused by vasoconstriction of the afferent arteriole, leading to a decrease in renal vascular tone.[4] Nephrotoxicity manifests as an increase in serum creatinine concentrations and, in some cases, increases in serum potassium and decreases in serum magnesium concentrations. The renal effects are related to the dose of cyclosporine and can be reversed within the first 6 months after transplant by lowering the dose of cyclosporine in many cases.[5] However, the effects of chronic cyclosporine use on the kidney after 6 months after transplant compromise long-term renal function in all organs and contribute to chronic allograft nephropathy (CAN) in kidney transplant recipients.[5] Nephrotoxicity of cyclosporine can be reduced by delaying administration after transplantation by using induction therapy with an IL-2 receptor antagonist or antilymphocyte globulin. Other strategies to reduce the risk of nephrotoxicity include diligent monitoring of cyclosporine concentrations, maintaining adequate hydration, and avoiding other nephrotoxic agents, such as amphotericin B, aminoglycosides, and nonsteroidal antiinflammatory agents.

Neurologic effects of cyclosporine can manifest as mild symptoms, such as tremors, headaches, insomnia, and peripheral neuropathy, but can be as severe as seizures. Neurologic toxicities are reported in 10% to 28% of patients receiving cyclosporine.[6] Similar to nephrotoxicity, the neurologic effects are related to the dose of cyclosporine and can be limited or reversed by lowering cyclosporine concentrations.

Other metabolic side effects of cyclosporine include hypertension, hyperlipidemia, and new-onset diabetes mellitus after transplant. Regimens that combine cyclosporine with steroids are associated with a higher incidence of hypertension, hyperlipidemia, and diabetes.[7,8] Hypertension is reported in as many as 80% of patients.[9] The primary mechanism by which cyclosporine causes hypertension is due to vasoconstriction of the afferent arteriole, which is accompanied by sodium and water retention.[10] The magnitude by which blood pressure increases is dependent on the dose of cyclosporine. Overall, blood pressure increases an average of 7 mm Hg in patients receiving cyclosporine, but ranges from 5 mm Hg in patients receiving low doses to 11 mm Hg in patients receiving high doses.[11] Diagnosis and treatment of hypertension are similar to those in the nontransplant population. Dihydropyridine calcium channel blockers (ie, nifedipine, amlodipine) were once considered to be the first-line drugs of choice because of their vasodilatory effects on the renal vasculature, which directly counterbalanced the effects of cyclosporine. More recent studies, however, failed to demonstrate any benefit of the calcium channel blockers over other antihypertensive agents, namely angiotensin-converting enzyme inhibitors.[12] Generally, 2 to 3 antihypertensives are necessary to adequately control blood pressure in transplant recipients.[13] Similarly, hyperlipidemia occurs in 60% to 70% of patients receiving cyclosporine.[14] The lipid profile has been correlated with cyclosporine levels.[15] Hyperlipidemia is often treated with 3-hydroxy-3-methyl-glutaryl-CoA (HMG-CoA) reductase inhibitors ("statins") to lower total cholesterol. Cyclosporine can cause hyperglycemia through its direct toxic effect on the islet cells of the pancreas, which decreases insulin production. However, the effects of cyclosporine on blood sugars are less pronounced than tacrolimus.[16]

Cosmetic side effects of cyclosporine can decrease the quality of life for transplant recipients. The most commonly reported cosmetic side effects associated with cyclosporine include gingival hyperplasia, acne, and hirsutism. Gingival hyperplasia is reported in 13% to 85% of transplant patients.[17] Acne is reported most commonly in adolescents, but is also common in adults.[18] Gingival hyperplasia and acne are best managed by good oral and skin hygiene, respectively. Hirsutism affects nearly 70% of patients taking cyclosporine and can be dose-related.[18]

Drug-drug interactions are common with cyclosporine because CYP 3A4 is a common pathway for many drug interactions. The most common medications known to alter cyclosporine metabolism are found in **Table 2**. The magnitude of drug interactions with cyclosporine can be profound, depending on the affinity of the co-administered drug. For example, diltiazem and erythromycin, inhibitors of CYP 3A4, can increase cyclosporine concentrations up to 82%.[19] Rifampin, on the other hand, is a potent inducer of CYP 3A4, and can decrease cyclosporine concentrations

Table 2				
Common drug interactions reported with immunosuppressive agents				
Cyclosporine, Tacrolimus, Sirolimus, Everolimus		**Mycophenolate Mofetil, Mycophenolic Acid**		**Azathioprine**
Increase	**Decrease**	**Increase**	**Decrease**	**Increase**
Cimetidine	Antacids	Acyclovir	Antacids	Allopurinol
Clarithromycin	(tacrolimus only)	Ganciclovir	Cholestyramine	Febuxostat
Diltiazem	Carbamazepine		Cyclosporine	
Erythromycin	Cholestyramine			
Fluconazole	Phenobarbital			
Grapefruit juice	Phenytoin			
Itraconazole	Rifampin			
Ketoconazole				
Levofloxacin				
Nefazodone				
Nicardipine				
Protease inhibitors				
Voriconazole				

by 50%.[20] When possible, it is best to avoid administering drugs known to alter CYP 3A4 metabolism, although the drug interaction can easily be managed by carefully monitoring cyclosporine concentrations. Cyclosporine is also a weak inhibitor of CYP 3A4 and can alter the metabolism of weaker substrates for the enzyme, such as the case for statins, the antihyperlipidemic medications. Cyclosporine can increase statin concentrations and toxicities, such as myopathies. When statins are indicated for hyperlipidemia in patients receiving cyclosporine, the drugs should be started at the lowest dose possible and titrated slowly for effect, while carefully monitoring for toxicities associated with the statin. Simvastatin is altered to the greatest extent and should be avoided with cyclosporine.

Administering cyclosporine with food decreases the amount and extent of cyclosporine absorption. When taken within 30 minutes of a high-fat meal (45 g fat), cyclosporine absorption decreases significantly, with peak concentrations approximately one-third of the concentrations reached when taken on an empty stomach.[21] It is important that the timing of cyclosporine administration be consistent with regards to meals to maintain stable cyclosporine concentrations. Grapefruit juice is a potent inhibitor of CYP 3A4 and increases cyclosporine concentrations by up to 55%, because of furocoumarins, such as quercetin, naringin, and bergamottin.[22]

Starting doses of cyclosporine range from 8 to 18 mg/kg per day, administered every 12 hours. In general, 3-drug regimens use lower starting doses, whereas 2-drug regimens use higher starting doses. Cyclosporine can be administered intravenously (IV) at one-third of the oral dose. The IV dose can be administered intermittently every 12 hours as a slow infusion over 4 to 6 hours or the total daily dose can be administered continuously over 24 hours. Typical IV doses of cyclosporine range from 2 to 5 mg/kg per day. Higher cyclosporine doses, 2- to 4-times adult doses, ranging from 14 to 18 mg/kg per day, are required for children to account for increased metabolism of the drug. It is imperative that cyclosporine concentrations are monitored to minimize the risk of toxicity and over-immunosuppression. The target cyclosporine concentration is dependent on the assay used, the type of transplant, concomitant immunosuppression, the time after transplant, and the transplant center. High-performance liquid chromatography (HPLC) is the preferred assay for cyclosporine because it measures only the parent compound. Target concentrations range from 100 to 300 ng/mL. Radioimmunoassay (RIA) measures both the parent compound and metabolites, resulting in target ranges approximately 20% to 25% higher than HPLC for cyclosporine levels. Peak concentration, known as C_2 monitoring, has been shown to correlate better with rejection within the first year after transplant. The suggested therapeutic range for C_2 concentrations varies based on the time after transplant: 1500 to 2000 ng/mL for the first 6 months and 700 to 900 ng/mL during months 6 to 12.[23]

Tacrolimus

Tacrolimus (Prograf®) binds to a cytoplasmic protein called FK-binding protein-12 (FKBP12). The tacrolimus-FKBP12 inhibits calineurin, similar to the cyclosporine-cyclophilin complex. The net result is the same effect as cyclosporine: inhibition of NF-AT activation of cytokine transcription, namely IL-2. Thus, tacrolimus and cyclosporine produce identical effects to disrupt the immune system and, therefore, should not be used simultaneously in the immunosuppressive regimen.

Absorption of tacrolimus is more consistent than cyclosporine, but averages only 30%. Peak concentrations are generally reached within 1 to 3 hours. Once absorbed, 99% of tacrolimus is bound to plasma proteins. The volume of distribution of tacrolimus is low, ranging from 0.8 to 1.9 L/kg. The half-life of tacrolimus ranges from 8 to 12 hours.

Akin to cyclosporine, tacrolimus has the dose-limiting side effects of nephrotoxicity and neurotoxicity (see **Table 1**). Tacrolimus also causes vasoconstriction of the afferent arteriole of the kidney, leading to the nephrotoxicity. Nephrotoxicity associated with tacrolimus also manifests with increases in serum creatinine concentrations. However, the effects of tacrolimus on the kidney result in more pronounced effects on electrolytes, namely hyperkalemia and hypomagnesemia. Similar to cyclosporine, early nephrotoxic effects can be reversed or prevented by reducing or delaying the dose of tacrolimus, but late effects are generally irreversible and can contribute to long-term renal dysfunction in all organs and CAN in kidney transplant recipients. Nephrotoxicity can be minimized by monitoring tacrolimus concentrations, maintaining adequate hydration, and avoiding administering other nephrotoxic agents.

Neurotoxicity associated with tacrolimus manifests in a similar manner to cyclosporine, ranging from tremors, insomnia, headaches, and peripheral neuropathy, to more serious seizure complications. Although the neurologic effects of tacrolimus are reported with similar frequency to cyclosporine (5–30%), the effects appear to be more pronounced and major neurologic complications are reported more frequently with tacrolimus.[6,24] Several studies also note improvement in neurologic complications after tacrolimus is switched to cyclosporine.[24,25]

The metabolic side effects of tacrolimus are similar to those of cyclosporine, but differ in incidence. Hypertension and hyperlipidemia are reported less frequently with tacrolimus-based regimens compared with cyclosporine-based regimens.[20,26] In one study, conversion from cyclosporine to tacrolimus resulted in reduction or resolution of hypertension in 59.1% of patients and hyperlipidemia in 63.5% of patients.[27] In contrast, tacrolimus appears to be associated with a higher incidence of diabetes after transplant than cyclosporine by decreasing insulin production through its direct nephrotoxic effects on the islet cells of the pancreas.[16] Treatment of diabetes after transplant involves oral hypoglycemic agents, such as sulfonylureas or insulin-sensitizing agents, or insulin, when oral agents do not provide adequate control. Decreasing tacrolimus levels does not appear to have any benefit in lowering blood glucose levels or reversing diabetes after transplant.[28] Tacrolimus is not associated with the same cosmetic side effects as cyclosporine. In fact, studies have demonstrated improvement or reversal of cosmetic side effects, including gingival hyperplasia and hirsutism.[27,29,30] However, tacrolimus can cause alopecia.[20]

Because tacrolimus is metabolized by CYP 3A4, drug-drug interactions are the same as those seen with cyclosporine (see **Table 2**), with similar magnitude. As with cyclosporine, co-administration of drugs known to interfere with tacrolimus metabolism should be avoided when possible, or tacrolimus concentrations should be carefully monitored. Tacrolimus is also a weak inhibitor of CYP 3A4 and can increase serum concentrations of weaker substates, such as the stains, but not to the same degree as cyclosporine. One drug interaction that is unique to tacrolimus occurs with concomitant administration of medications that contain positive cations, such as calcium-, magnesium- and aluminum-containing antacids, sodium bicarbonate, and magnesium oxide. These medications bind to tacrolimus in the GI tract and decrease overall tacrolimus absorption.[31] This interaction can be easily managed by separating the dosing time of the antacids from tacrolimus by at least 2 hours. The same interaction does not occur with cyclosporine.

Comparable with cyclosporine, administration of tacrolimus with food decreases the absorption of tacrolimus. High-fat meals further decrease the rate and extent of tacrolimus absorption from the GI tract by up to 27%.[32] Consistent timing of tacrolimus administration related to meals is important to minimize fluctuations in tacrolimus concentrations. Grapefruit juice can also interact with tacrolimus via irreversible inhibition of CYP 3A4 enzymes.[22]

Initial starting doses of tacrolimus range from 0.1 to 0.3 mg/kg/d administered every 12 hours. Tacrolimus can also be administered IV as a continuous infusion over 24 hours. The IV doses are one-third the oral doses, with usual doses ranging from 0.05 to 0.1 mg/k/d. Trough tacrolimus concentrations correlate well with rejection and toxicity and should be closely monitored through the duration of therapy. Trough concentrations should be measured immediately before the next dose of tacrolimus is administered. Whole blood concentrations are generally monitored via RIA, which measures both parent drug and metabolites, or HPLC, which measures parent drug only; target ranges for tacrolimus will be lower for the latter assay. The target range for tacrolimus concentrations varies with the time after transplantation, the immunosuppressive regimen, and the transplant type. Generally, target ranges are 15 to 20 ng/mL within the first month after transplantation, 10 to 15 ng/mL for the next 3 months, and 5 to 12 ng/mL after month 3 after transplant.[20] Serum concentrations should be measured multiple times weekly immediately after transplant and can be monitored less frequently as organ function stabilizes and the time after transplant increases.

CORTICOSTEROIDS

Corticosteroids are the most widely used of all the immunosuppressants and have been used since the first solid organ transplants were performed. They continue to be a key part of the immunosuppressive regimen, even though they are associated with multiple side effects. The most commonly used corticosteroids in transplantation are methylprednisolone and prednisone.

Corticosteroids are nonspecific in their immunosuppressive action. They block multiple co-signaling cytokines that are responsible for interlymphocytic communications. Specifically, corticosteroids block the synthesis of IL-1, -2, -3, and -6, interferon-γ, and tumor necrosis factor α. As a result, corticosteroids interfere with cell migration, recognition, and cytotoxic effects.

Once absorbed, prednisone is converted to prednisolone, which has multiple effects in the body. Because prednisone is well absorbed from the GI tract and has a long biological half-life, it is generally dosed once daily. High dose are divided multiple times throughout the day to improve patient tolerability.

Adverse effects are common with high doses of corticosteroids, affecting up to 10% of patients, and range from hyperglycemia, insomnia, mood changes, and increased appetite (see **Table 1**). Less common side effects are generally seen with prolonged doses and include cataracts, hirsutism, bruising, acne, sodium and water retention, hypertension, osteoporosis, and esophagitis. In children, corticosteroids are known to decrease growth and development, both physically and cognitively.[33]

Corticosteroids are metabolized by the CYP 3A4 enzyme system and, therefore, are subject to drug interactions. However, given that corticosteroids are either used in high doses or in combination with other immunosuppressives, the drug interactions prove to be clinically insignificant. Some drugs known to decrease corticosteroid exposure are the barbiturates phenytoin and rifampin.

During the perioperative period, high doses of corticosteroids, specifically methylprednisone, are generally given for most immunosuppressive regimens. Doses are quickly tapered over the first few days after transplant and switched to oral agents, namely prednisone or prednisolone. Once patients are receiving daily doses of corticosteroids, it is preferable to administer the doses between 7 AM and 8 AM to mimic natural circadian rhythms of cortisol release within the body. For most immunosuppressive regimens, prednisone doses are tapered progressively over the course of the next few weeks to months, depending on organ function. In many cases, corticosteroids may be withdrawn completely within the first 6 to 12 months. Most immunosuppressive regimens limit the long-term use of corticosteroids. Many protocols use a steroid-withdrawal protocol, whereby corticosteroids are withdrawn within the first 1 to 6 months after transplant. At a minimum, most protocols aim to reduce corticosteroids to physiologic doses (equivalent of prednisone 5 mg daily doses) within the first 3 to 6 months after transplantation. It is important to remember that corticosteroids should never be discontinued abruptly, but slowly tapered over the course of several days to months, depending on the duration of therapy, to avoid suppression of the hypothalamic-pituitary-adrenal axis.

Corticosteroids are also used as the first-line agents for the treatment of acute rejection. Generally, treatment consists of high doses of IV methylprednisolone, 500 to 1000 mg, administered over 1 to 3 days. High doses of oral prednisone (200 mg) have also been administered for treatment of acute rejection, which are quickly tapered over 5 to 7 days.

ANTIMETABOLITES

Similar to corticosteroids, antimetabolites have been used since the early days of transplantation to inhibit proliferation of lymphocytes. The "gold standard" of immunosuppressive regimens has included azathioprine, along with corticosteroids and cyclosporine. However, it is recognized more recently that the newer agents have increased efficacy over this traditional regimen. Today, newer antimetabolite agents, such as mycophenolic acid, continue to be a key part of the immunosuppressive regimen.

Mycophenolate Mofetil and Mycophenolate Sodium

Mycophenolic acid (MPA) was fist isolated from the *Penicillin glaucum* mold. Currently, there are 2 formulations of MPA available: mycophenolate mofetil (Cellcept®), which is a pro-drug of MPA, commercially available as mycophenolate sodium, an enteric-coated, delayed release formulation (Myfortic®).

MPA exerts its immunosuppressive effect by inhibiting inosine monophosphate dehydrogenase (IMPDH), an enzyme responsible for the synthesis of the nucleotide guanosine. This enzyme is only used in the de novo pathway of nucleotide synthesis. Inhibition of IMPDH results in a reduction of DNA polymerase activity, which decreases lymphocyte proliferation. It is important to note that T and B lymphocytes depend only on the de novo pathway for nucleotide synthesis and do not have a salvage pathway to produce guanosine, unlike most other cells within the body. This makes MPA very specific in its actions, targeting primarily T and B lymphocytes, which decreases its overall effects on other cells in the body, thereby decreasing side effects to a great extent.

Mycophenolate mofetil serves as a pro-drug that helps to overcome degradation of MPA in the acid environment of the stomach. Mycophenolate mofetil is readily absorbed from the GI tract and is rapidly converted to MPA by first-pass metabolism. Absolute bioavailability of mycophenolate mofetil is 94%, and MPA concentrations reach peak levels within 1 hour after the dose of mycophenolate mofetil is administered. The commercially available mycophenolic acid formulation is enteric-coated to protect the drug from the acidic pH in the stomach and is absorbed from the upper portion of the small intestines. The absolute bioavailability of MPA is somewhat less than mycophenolate mofetil at 72%. Once absorbed, 97% of MPA is bound to albumin in the bloodstream. The volume of distribution of MPA is approximately 4 L/kg. The drug undergoes glucuronidation in the liver to form an inactive metabolite, mycophenolic acid glucuronide (MPAG). The half-life of MPA is 18 hours.

The most common adverse effects of MPA are related to its direct antiproliferative effects on the GI tract, leading to nausea, vomiting, abdominal pain, and diarrhea (see **Table 1**). Decreasing the dose or dividing the dose over more frequent dosing intervals (ie, 3 to 4 doses daily) can decrease the GI side effects associated with MPA. High doses of MPA can suppress the bone marrow, leading to leukopenia, thrombocytopenia, and anemia. It is important to note that because MPA alters DNA synthesis through inhibition of nucleotide synthesis, MPA is teratogenic and should be avoided in patients who are pregnant. The Pregnancy Category of MPA was recently changed to Category D, indicating the risks outweigh benefits of taking the drug.

Co-administration of magnesium- or aluminum-containing antacids or cholestyramine can decrease the absorption of MPA (see **Table 2**). To avoid this drug interaction, doses should be separated by at least 2 hours from the MPA dose. Acyclovir, and presumably ganciclovir, competes with tubular secretion of MPAG, which can then be recycled back into the bloodstream, thereby increasing the immunosuppressive effects and toxicities associated with MPA. Cyclosporine can interfere with the enterohepatic recirculation of MPAG, decreasing MPA concentrations.[34] It may be necessary to administer higher doses of MPA with cyclosporine-based regimens, compared with tacrolimus. Conversely, tacrolimus-MPA–based regimens may be associated with more MPA toxicity, namely GI-related reactions.

Food can affect the time to reach peak concentrations and time to elimination of the drug. As a result, overall exposure to MPA, reflected as the area-under-the-curve (AUC), is unaltered when MPA is administered with food. Therefore, patients experiencing GI-related side effects may be told to take MPA with food to increase tolerability.

Mycophenolate mofetil is available in multiple formulations, including oral capsules and tablets, an oral suspension, and an IV formulation. Although the two are not considered to be bioequivalent, oral and IV doses can be administered at the same doses.[35] Mycophenolate sodium is only available in oral tablets. Doses of MPA are based on the type of organ transplant. Cardiac transplantation generally requires a higher degree of immunosuppression, warranting higher starting doses of MPA. Starting doses of mycophenolate mofetil are 1500 mg twice daily for cardiac transplants and 1000 mg twice daily for all other organ transplants. Because mycophenolate sodium does not contain the mofetil ester, starting doses are smaller at 1440 mg twice daily for cardiac transplants and 720 mg twice daily for all other transplants. Plasma MPA concentrations can be measured, although the clinical utility is somewhat debatable. Monitoring AUC levels, which requires measurement of 2 to 4 sequential MPA concentrations, correlates best with rejection, but not with toxicity.[36] The reported reference range for MPA AUC levels is 30 to 60 mcg/mL/h.[37] Trough MPA concentrations do not correlate well with rejection, but are the most commonly use method to monitor MPA because of the ease of blood sampling for a single measurement.[36]

Azathioprine

Azathioprine itself is an inactive compound that must be converted to 6-mercapto-purine (6-MP) in the blood. 6-MP is metabolized by hypoxanthine-guanine phospho-ribosyltransferase to active metabolites, 6-thioguanine nucleotides (TGNs). TGNs are incorporated into the nucleic acids, which block both the de novo and salvage pathways of nucleic acid synthesis. Ultimately, azathioprine disrupts DNA, RNA, and protein synthesis within the cell, thereby blocking cell proliferation.

Azathioprine is well absorbed after oral dosing and approximately 47% is converted to 6-MP after absorption. Protein binding is approximately 30% for both azathioprine and 6-MP. The volume of distribution of azathioprine is 0.8 L/kg. 6-MP is metabolized by xanthine oxidase (XO), found in the liver and GI tract, to the final end product, 6-thiouric acid, which is excreted by the kidneys. The half-life of azathio-prine, the parent compound, is 3 hours, whereas the half-life of 6-MP is approximately 60 to 90 minutes. However, the active metabolites, the TGNs, have a much longer half-life, estimated to be up to 9 days.[38]

The adverse effects of azathioprine are related to the disruption of both the de novo and salvage pathways of nucleotide production. The resulting effects on DNA, RNA, and protein synthesis are evident in all cells within the body and are not limited to T and B lymphocytes. The dose-limiting toxicity is bone marrow suppres-sion, which is related to the dose of azathioprine (see **Table 1**). Other adverse reactions reported to azathioprine result from its effects on blocking proliferation of other cells. Nausea, vomiting, and abdominal pain result from the effects of azathio-prine on cells in the GI tract. Similarly, azathioprine affects hair follicles and can cause alopecia. Hepatotoxicity and pancreatitis are reported less commonly with azathio-prine. The occurrence of all adverse effects is related to the dose of azathioprine and is reversible by lowering or discontinuing the drug. Because azathioprine disrupts cell proliferation of many cell lines, it is teratogenic (Pregnancy Category D) and its use should be avoided in pregnant women.

The most significant drug interaction with azathioprine occurs with drugs that inhibit the activity of XO, namely allopurinol and febuxostat (see **Table 2**). Allopurinol can increase azathioprine and 6-MP concentrations by as much as 4-fold.[39] Blocking XO shifts the metabolism of azathioprine and 6-MP to favor production of TGNs, the pharmacologically active metabolites which, in turn, increases suppression of cell proliferation. The net result is increased bone marrow suppression and pancytope-nia.[39] When allopurinol or febuxostat are co-administered with azathioprine, the dose of azathioprine should be reduced by 50% to 75% to avoid toxicities. Other drug interactions with azathioprine result from administration of drugs with overlapping bone marrow suppression or GI toxicities, such as sulfamethoxazole-trimethoprim, ganciclovir, and sirolimus.

Initial starting doses of azathioprine are 3 to 5 mg/kg administered as a single daily dose. Therapeutic drug monitoring does not target azathioprine or 6-MP concentrations, but rather the dose-limiting toxicity of blood cell production, namely white blood cell (WBC) count. The goal for azathioprine therapy is to maintain the WBC count between 3500 and 6000 cells/mm^3. When initiating therapy, WBC count should be monitored frequently to avoid oversuppression of the bone marrow. Thus, patients are usually instructed to take azathioprine doses in the evening to allow for dose adjustments based on WBC counts.

PROLIFERATION SIGNAL INHIBITORS

The newest class of immunosuppressive agents, also known as mTOR inhibitors, targets the mammalian target of rapamycin (mTOR). These agents are often used as adjunctive therapy to reduce the dose of calcineurin inhibitors in an attempt to spare the long-term renal effects.

Sirolimus

The first Federal Drug Administration–approved agent in the class of mTOR inhibitors is sirolimus (Rapamune®), also known as rapamycin. Sirolimus is an immunosuppressive macrolide antibiotic that is structurally similar to tacrolimus. Resembling tacrolimus, sirolimus binds to FKBP12. However, the resulting sirolimus-FKBP12 complex does not inhibit calcineurin and cytokine production. Instead the complex binds to a regulatory kinase, mTOR, which inhibits the cellular response to cytokines. Specifically, sirolimus inhibits stimulation of mTOR by IL-2, IL-4, and IL-15, preventing activation of kinases that advance the cell cycle from the G$_1$ to the S phase. Therefore, the ultimate action of sirolimus is to inhibit cytokine-mediated progression of the cell cycle in response to IL-2, thereby inhibiting T-lymphocyte proliferation.

Sirolimus is poorly absorbed from the GI tract, with only 27% bioavailability with the tablet formulation and 15% bioavailability with the oral solution. Peak concentrations are reached within 1 to 2 hours after oral administration. After absorption, 92% of sirolimus is bound to plasma proteins. Sirolimus is widely distributed in the body because of the presence of FKBP12 in red blood cells (RBCs), resulting in a volume of distribution of 12 L/kg. Similar to tacrolimus, sirolimus is also metabolized in the liver and GI tract by the CYP 3A4 enzyme system and PGP. However, the half-life of sirolimus is much longer, approximately 62 hours. In patients with liver dysfunction, the half-life can be as long as 110 hours.[40]

Thrombocytopenia is evident within the first 2 weeks starting sirolimus therapy but improves as treatment is continued (see **Table 1**). Leukopenia and anemia may be transient.[41] Bone marrow suppression appears to be dose related as thrombocytopenia and leukopenia correlate with sirolimus concentrations above 15 ng/mL.[42] Sirolimus is associated with dyslipidemia, specifically hypercholesterolemia and hypertriglyceridemia. The mechanism may be related to an overproduction of lipoproteins or inhibition of lipoprotein lipase.[43] Cholesterol and triglyceride levels peak within the first 3 months after starting sirolimus, but decrease after 1 year of therapy. Hyperlipidemia can be managed by decreasing the dose or discontinuing sirolimus, or starting a statin or fibric acid derivative. Despite the high levels of cholesterol and triglycerides, this does not appear to be a major risk factor for cardiovascular complications within the first year of transplant.[43] Sirolimus causes proteinuria, which appears to be dose-related.[44] There are conflicting reports about the significance of the proteinuria causing kidney damage. Angiotensin converting enzyme (ACE) inhibitors may help to control sirolimus-induced proteinuria.[44] Siroli-mus inhibits smooth muscle proliferation and intimal thickening, which prolongs wound healing and can lead to wound dehiscence.[45] Mouth ulcers are reported more commonly with sirolimus oral solution, although they can occur with the tablet formulation as well, and may be the result of herpes simplex reactivation.[46] Reversible interstitial pneumonitis has been described.[40] Other adverse effects that have been reported with sirolimus include increased liver enzymes, hypertension, rash, diarrhea, acne, and arthralgias. The combination of sirolimus and a calcineurin inhibitor may have a synergistic effect on nephrotoxicity early after kidney transplant.[47]

Because of CYP 3A4 metabolism, sirolimus is prone to numerous drug interactions, comparable with cyclosporine and tacrolimus (see **Table 2**). Cyclo-sporine increases sirolimus concentrations; conversely, sirolimus also increases cyclosporine concentrations because of competitive inhibition of CYP 3A4 and PGP. The doses of each drug should be separated by at least 4 hours, and lower doses of each should be used to avoid toxicities of both drugs. Tacrolimus does not produce the same results.

Food decreases sirolimus absorption, particularly when administered with a high-fat meal. Total sirolimus exposure is reduced by 23% to 35% after a high-fat meal. Grapefruit juice also inhibits the metabolism of sirolimus, leading to increased concentrations.

Sirolimus is approved with a fixed-dose regimen, using a 6-mg or 15-mg loading dose, followed by 2 mg or 5 mg, respectively. However, therapeutic drug monitoring is advocated to maintain adequate immunosuppression and avoid toxicities. Siroli-mus concentrations should be measured in whole blood using HPCL, which mea-sures the parent compound only. Target levels are 10 to 15 ng/mL when used in combination with a calcineurin inhibitor, or 15 to 20 ng/mL when not used in combination with a calcineurin inhibitor. RIA, which measures both parent compound and metabolites, can also be used to measure sirolimus concentrations, but higher target levels should be used with reference ranges of 15 to 20 ng/mL and 20 to 30 ng/mL, respectively.

Everolimus

Everolimus (Zortress®) is a new immunosuppressive agent approved in the United States, although it has been available for several years in Europe. Resembling sirolimus, everolimus binds to FKBP12 to form a complex that binds to mTOR, preventing IL-2–mediated T-lymphocyte proliferation. Approximately 74% of the drug is bound to plasma proteins after oral absorption. The volume of distribution is variable in kidney transplant recipients, ranging from 107 to 342 L, likely reflecting distribution to FKBP12 receptors in RBC. Everolimus is metabolized by CYP 3A4 and PGP in the GI tract and liver. The half-life of everolimus appears to be shorter than sirolimus at 30 hours.

Adverse reactions reported with everolimus appear to be similar to sirolimus. Everolimus delays wound healing because of the antiproliferative effects on smooth muscle. Hyperlipidemia is also common with everolimus. Everolimus also causes proteinuria, which has been reported to increase the incidence of nephrotoxicity in cyclosporine-based regimens. Leukopenia, anemia, and thrombocytopenia are re-ported, although there are no data to compare the incidence with sirolimus. Other adverse reactions reported with everolimus include peripheral edema, constipation, hypertension, nausea, and urinary tract infections.[48]

Drug interactions with everolimus are similar to those seen with cyclosporine, tacrolimus, and sirolimus. Single dose studies indicate everolimus concentrations are increased by concomitant administration of cyclosporine, ketoconazole, erythromycin, and verapamil, whereas rifampin decreases everolimus concentrations. Grapefruit juice also increases everolimus concentrations, whereas a high-fat meal decreases concentrations by 60%.[48]

Everolimus therapy should be initiated at 0.75 mg twice daily. Doses should be adjusted to maintain trough concentrations between 3 and 8 ng/mL.[49]

Belatacept

Belatacept (Nulojix®) is the newest immunosuppressive agent approved in the United States. Unlike the other maintenance immunosuppressants, which are oral medications, belatacept is an IV medication. Belatacept is a costimulation blocker that binds to CD80 and CD86 ligands found on antigen presenting cells (APCs). Blockade of CD80 and CD86 prevents interaction with the CD28 receptor, a critical costimulatory receptor found on T lymphocytes responsible for activation of naïve T lymphocytes after presentation of antigens via APCs.[50] Such T lymphocytes that do not receive a costimulatory signal become anergic and undergoes apoptosis.[51]

Side effects of belatacept include anemia, diarrhea, peripheral edema, hypertension, dyslipidemia, potassium abnormalities, and leukopenia. The most serious adverse effect associated with belatacept is post-transplant lymphoproliferative disorder (PTLD), seen most commonly in patients without immunity to Epstein-Barr virus (EBV).[52] Belatacept is contraindicated in patients who are EBV seronegative. Progressive multifactoral leukoencephalopathy (PML) has also been reported in clinical trials with belatacept. The starting dose of belatacept is 10 mg/kg on the day of transplantation, 4 days after transplantation, and 2, 4, 8 and 12 weeks after transplantation. Beginning 16 weeks after the transplant, maintenance doses of 5 mg/kg should be administered every 4 weeks. Basiliximab should be given as induction therapy before starting maintenance therapy with belatacept in combination with mycophenolate mofetil and prednisone. Belatacept may have a role in preserving kidney function in kidney transplant patients who are at risk for chronic allograft nephropathy.[52]

LYMPHOCYTE-DEPLETING AGENTS

Certain polyclonal and monoclonal antibodies that target T or B lymphocytes can cause lymphocyte depletion of one or both cell lines. These agents are useful for induction therapy administered before transplantation to provide a high degree of immunosuppression at the time of transplantation or as treatment for acute cellular rejection to reverse the effects of the activated immune system on the transplanted organ.

Antithymocyte Globulin

The antithymocyte globulins are polyclonal antibodies that target thymocytes (T cells). The 2 currently available preparations are ATG (ATGAM®), an equine preparation, and RATG (Thymoglobulin®), a rabbit preparation. Because the rabbit preparation is more potent than ATG and better tolerated because of lower immunogenicity, it is the primary agent used today for transplantation.[53] The products are prepared by injecting human T lymphocytes into an animal medium (horses for ATG and rabbits for RATG). The animals produce an immunologic response to the human cells, generating antibodies directed at antigens expressed on the human T lymphocytes. The antibodies are removed from the serum of the animals, purified, and pasteurized into the respective products for use in humans. The result is a polyclonal antibody product that targets a number of receptors found on lymphocytes, including CD2, CD3, CD4,

CD8, CD25, and CD45, as well as others. Upon binding to the various receptors, the drugs cause a complement-mediated cell lysis, which ultimately results in lymphocyte depletion. Damaged T lymphocytes are subsequently removed by the spleen, liver, and lungs. Because some of the target receptors are not exclusive to T lymphocytes, other cells are also affected by administration of the antithymocyte globulins, including B lymphocytes, WBC, RBC, and platelets.

Both ATG and RATG bind primarily to circulating T lymphocytes in the bloodstream and are poorly distributed into lymphoid tissue in the body. The volume of distribution for RATG is 0.12 L/kg. The terminal half-life differs for the 2 products: 5.7 days for ATG and 30 days for RATG. Antibodies can form to the animal serum after administration of these products. Antiequine antibodies form in 78% of patients receiving ATG, and antirabbit antibodies form in 68% of patients receiving RATG. The clinical significance of the respective antibodies is not well understood.

The side effects of ATG and RATG are related to the lack of specificity of the polyclonal antibodies for T lymphocytes. Pancytopenia can occur after therapy because of direct lysis of the other circulating blood cells. This often limits the number of doses and duration of therapy for these products. Other side effects are related to the immune reaction that occurs with the infusion of the antibody products that can result in anaphylaxis or severe cytokine-release syndrome, manifesting as fever, hypotension, hypertension, tachycardia, dyspnea, urticaria, and rash. Patients must be monitored closely when receiving ATG or RATG throughout the infusion. A rapid rate of infusion is associated with a higher incidence of cytokine-release syndrome and severe reactions. The infusion-related reactions can be minimized or prevented by administering acetaminophen, diphenhydramine, and corticosteroids before starting the infusion. Serum sickness can occur after administration of ATG because of the equine nature of the product; serum sickness can also occur with RATG but is rare.

The immune response to live vaccines can be altered by the administration of ATG and RATG. Live vaccines should be avoided within 2 months of receiving either product, if possible.

Both ATG and RATG are available as IV formulations only. The dosing of ATG is 10 to 30 mg/kg per day as a single dose. RATG is administered at doses of 1 to 1.5 mg/kg per day as a single dose. The duration of therapy depends on the indication of the product. Induction therapy generally involves 5 to 7 days of therapy, whereas treatment of acute cellular rejection requires 7 to 14 days of therapy. Premedication with acetaminophen, diphenhydramine, and corticosteroids should be administered 30 to 60 minutes before each dose of ATG or RATG. Both products should be administered via central line or high-flow vein whenever possible. RATG has been administered peripherally with the addition of hydrocortisone (20 mg) and heparin (1000 U) to reduce the risk of phlebitis and thrombosis.[54]

Alemtuzumab

Alemtuzumab (Campath-1H®) is a humanized monoclonal antibody directed against CD52, produced through recombinant DNA technology in Chinese hamster ovary cells. The CD52 target is found on several immune cells, including T and B lymphocytes, macrophages, monocytes, eosinophils, and natural killer cells. Alemtuzumab is approved for use in B-lymphocyte chronic lymphocytic leukemia (B-CLL), but is also used for solid organ transplantation. Upon binding to the CD52 receptor, alemtuzumab binds to T and B lymphocytes in the blood, bone marrow, lymphatic system, and organs, causing rapid, complete, and long-lasting lymphocyte depletion.

B lymphocytes return within a few months, but T lymphocytes do not fully recover for 1 to 3 years after alemtuzumab therapy.[55]

Although the pharmacokinetics of alemtuzumab has not been formally studied in solid organ transplantation, data from its use in B-CLL indicate that the volume of distribution is 0.18 L/kg after repeated dosing. The half-life is reported as 11 hours after the first 30-mg dose after rapid dose escalation. The same pharmacokinetic parameters may not apply to solid organ transplantation, however, as the dosing strategies are different for the 2 indications.

Adverse effects associated with alemtuzumab include severe infusion-related reactions, which manifest as rigors, hypotension, fever, dyspnea, brochospasms, and chills. Administration of acetaminophen, diphenhydramine, and corticosteroids helps to lessen, although not completely eliminate, these effects. Hematologic reactions, including neutropenia, lymphopenia, thrombocytopenia, and anemia, are reported frequently with alemtuzumab.

Alemtuzumab is most commonly administered as a single 30-mg dose in solid organ transplantation, without dose escalation, IV over 2 hours. The same dose is used for both induction therapy and for treatment of acute cellular rejection. Other dosing strategies that have been used in solid organ transplantation include 0.3 mg/kg per dose for one or more doses, and two 20-mg doses administered on the day of transplant and the first postoperative day.[56]

Acetaminophen, diphenhydramine, and corticosteroids must be administered 30 to 60 minutes before infusion. Vital signs must be closely monitored immediately after the infusion.

Muromonab-CD3

Muromonab-CD3, also known as OKT3 (Orthoclone OKT3®), was the first monoclonal antibody approved for use in the United States. OKT3 targets the CD3 receptor found exclusively on mature T lymphocytes. The antibody is a murine-derived antibody that causes complete and rapid T-lymphocyte lysis and depletion. Because of its potency and specificity for T lymphocytes, OKT3 was used extensively as induction therapy and as treatment of allograft rejection. However, OKT3 is associated with significant side effects due to the profound cytokine release, which led to fever, chills, rigors, pruritus, and alterations in blood pressure, capillary leak syndrome and pulmonary edema.[57] The effects were most pronounced with the first dose, and were best managed by prophylactic administration of acetaminophen, diphenhydramine, and corticosteroids before OKT3. With the discovery of newer antibodies that were better tolerated and resulted in equivalent or better outcomes, OKT3 eventually became the last-line treatment for resistant rejection episodes. Because use of OKT3 declined, the manufacturer discontinued the drug from the market in 2010.

NON-LYMPHOCYTE–DEPLETING ANTIBODIES
Basiliximab

Basiliximab (Simulect) is a chimeric, murine-derived, monoclonal antibody directed at CD25, expressed on activated T lymphocytes. Daclizumab (Zenapax) is a similar drug with a humanized chimeric structure in the same class, known as IL-2 receptor antagonists, but was removed from the market in 2009. Both drugs exert the same mechanism of action. Upon binding to the receptor, basiliximab competitively blocks IL-2 to prevent activation and proliferation of T lymphocytes. Basiliximab has a volume of distribution of 8 L and saturates CD25 immediately after administration. The terminal half-life of basiliximab is approximately 7 days. Liver transplant recipients may require an additional dose of basiliximab if more than 10 L of ascites is removed after transplantation because clearance of basiliximab is increased with drainage of ascites.[58]

Few adverse reactions have been reported with the IL-2 receptor antagonists. Basiliximab is not associated infusion-related reactions, unlike the depleting antibodies. The dose of basiliximab is a fixed dose of 20 mg administered intravenously on the day of transplant and 4 days after transplant. The dose is administered as a slow infusion over 20 to 30 minutes.

INVESTIGATIONAL AGENTS FOR SOLID ORGAN TRANSPLANTATION
Bortezomib

Bortezomib is a proteosomal inhibitor currently approved for use in multiple myeloma marketed as Velcade. Bortezomib binds to the 26S proteosome responsible for degradation of regulatory molecules critical for various cellular mechanisms, including protein synthesis, cell cycle, transcription and signaling, immune response, and antigen presentation. The result is arrest of the cell cycle and subsequent apoptosis. Bortezomib appears to have a specific effect on antibody-producing plasma cells and has been used in solid organ transplantation for the treatment of antibody-mediated rejection and reduction of donor-specific antibody (DSA) levels.[59] The most commonly reported side effects of bortezomib include GI effects and thrombocytopenia. Paresthesias have been reported rarely.

Rituximab

Rituximab (Rituxan) is a humanized monoclonal antibody against the CD20 receptor found on B lymphocytes. Rituximab is currently approved for CD20-positive non-Hodgkins lymphoma, CD20-positive CLL, and rheumatoid arthritis. Upon binding to the CD20 receptor, rituximab induced complement-mediated B lymphocyte lysis. Rituximab has been used in transplantation for treatment of CD20-positive PTLD, antibody-mediated rejection, and reduction of DSA before transplantation.[60-62] Adverse reactions include infusion-related reactions resulting in urticaria, hypotension, angioedema, bronchospasm, pulmonary edema, and anaphylaxis.

SUMMARY

The multitude of immunosuppressants available for solid organ transplantation allows for many combinations of immunosuppressive therapies that can be tailored to a patient's specific lifestyle and immunosuppression needs. Newer agents currently being studied offer even more possibilities for the future to further reduce the incidence of acute rejection and prolong graft and patient survival.

REFERENCES

1. Najarian JS, Fryd DS, Strand M, et al. A single institution, randomized, prospective trial of cyclosporine versus azathioprine-antilymphocyte globulin for immunosuppression in renal allograft recipients. Ann Surg 1985;201:142–57.
2. 2008 Annual Report of the U. S. Organ Procurement and Transplantation Network and the Scientific Registry of Transplant Recipients: Transplant Data 1998–2007. Rockville, MD; U.S. Department of Health and Human Services, Health Resources and Services Administration, Healthcare Systems Bureau, Division of Transplantation.
3. First MR, Schroeder TJ, Monaco AP, et al. Cyclosporine bioavailability: dosing implications and impact on clinical outcomes in select transplantation subpopulations. Clin Transplant 1996;10:55–9.
4. Pradhan M, Leonard MG, Bridges ND, et al. Decline in renal function following thoracic organ transplantation in children. Am J Transplant 2002;2:652–7.

5. Nankivell BJ, Borrows RJ, Fung CLS, et al. Calcineurin inhibitor nephrotoxicity: longitudinal assessment by protocol histology. Transplantation 2004;78(4):557–65.
6. Bechstein WO. Neurotoxicity of calcineurin inhibitors: impact and clinical management. Transpl Int 2000;13:313–26.
7. Lladó L, Xiol X, Figueras J, et al. Immunosuppression without steroids in liver transplantations safe and reduced infection and metabolic complications: results from a prospective multicenter randomized study. J Hepatol 2006;44(4):710–6.
8. Veenstra CL, Best JH, Hornberg J, et al. Incidence of long-term cost of steroid-related side effects after renal transplantation. Am J Kidney Dis 1999;2:829.
9. Cifková R, Hallen H. Cyclosporine-induced hypertension. J Hyperten 2001;19(12):2283–5.
10. Büscher R, Vester U, Wingen AM, et al. Pathomechanisms and the diagnosis of arterial hypertension in pediatric renal allograft recipients. Pediatr Nephrol 2004;19:1201–11.
11. Robert N, Wong GWK, Wright JM. Effect of cyclosporine on blood pressure. Cochrane Database Syst Rev 2010;1:CD007893.
12. Midtvedt K, Hartmann A, Foss A, et al. Sustained improvement of renal graft function for two years in hypertensive renal transplant recipients treated with nifedipine as compared to lisinopril. Transplantation 2001;72(11):1787–92.
13. Malyszko J, Malyszko J, Bachórzewska-Gajewska H, et al. Inadequate blood pressure control in most kidney transplant recipients and patients with coronary artery disease with and without complications. Transplant Proc 2009;41:3069–72.
14. Marcén R. Immunosuppressive drugs in kidney transplantation. Drugs 2009;69(16): 2227–43.
15. Soylu A, Kavukçu S, Türkmen MA, et al. Correlation of C_0 and C_2 levels with lipid profiles in adolescent renal transplant recipients in the early and late posttransplant periods. Transplant Proc 2006;38(5):1286–9.
16. Vincenti F, Friman S, Scheuermann E, et al. Results of an international, randomized trial comparing glucose metabolism disorders and outcome with cyclosporine versus tacrolimus. Am J Transplant 2007;7(6):1506–14.
17. Wirnsberger GH, Pfranger R, Maurio A, et al. Effect of antibiotic treatment with azithromycin on cyclosporine A-induced gingival hyperplasia among renal transplant recipients. Transplant Proc 1998;30:2117–9.
18. Fortina AB, Piaserico S, Alaibac M, et al. Skin disorders in patients transplanted in childhood. Transplant Int 2005;18:360–5.
19. Martin JE, Daoud AJ, Schroeder TJ, et al. Pharmacoeconomics 1999;15(4):317-37.
20. Scott LJ, McKeage K, Keam SJ, et al. Tacrolimus: a further update of its use in the management of organ transplantation. Drugs 2003;63:1247–97.
21. Neoral® (cyclosporine, USP [MODIFIED]). Product Information. Novartis Pharmaceuticals Corporation, East Hanover, NJ, 2009.
22. Nowack R. Cytochrome P450 enzyme, and transport protein mediated herb-drug interactions in renal transplant patients: grapefruit juice, St. John's Wort – and beyond! Nephrol 2008;13:337–47.
23. Schiff J, Cole E, Cantarovich M. Therapeutic monitoring of calcineurin inhibitors for the nephrologists. Clin J Am Soc Nephrol 2007;2(2):374–84.
24. McDiarmid SV, Busuttil RW, Ascher NL, et al. FK506 (tacrolimus) compared with cyclosporine for primary immunosuppression after pediatric liver transplantation: results from the U.S. Multicenter Trial. Transplantation 1995;59(4):530–6.
25. Emre S, Genyk Y, Schluger LK, et al. Treatment of tacrolimus-related adverse effects by conversion to cyclosporine in liver transplant recipients. Transpl Int 2000;13:73–8.
26. Bowman LJ, Brennan DC. The role of tacrolimus in renal transplantation. Expert Opin Pharmacother 2008;9:635–43.

27. Margreiter R, Pohanka E, Sparacino V, et al. Open prospective multicenter study of conversion to tacrolimus therapy in renal transplant patients experiencing ciclosporin-related side-effects. Transpl Int 2005;18(7):816–23.

28. Paolillo JA, Boyle GJ, Law YM, et al. Posttransplant diabetes mellitus in pediatric thoracic organ recipients receiving tacrolimus-based immunosuppression. Transplantation 2001;71(2):252–6.

29. Reyes H, Jain A, Mazariegos G, et al. Long-term results after conversion from cyclosporine to tacrolimus in pediatric liver transplantation for acute and chronic rejection. Transplantation 2000;69(12):2573–80.

30. Busque S, Demers P, St-Louis G, et al. Conversion from Neoral (cyclosporine) to tacrolimus of kidney transplant recipients for gingival hyperplasia or hypertrichosis. Transpl Proc 1998;30:2117–9.

31. Chisholm MA, Mulloy LL, Jagadeesan M, et al. Coadministration of tacrolimus with anti-acid drugs. Transplantation 2003;76:665–6.

32. Staatz CE, Tett SE. Clinical pharmacokinetics and pharmacodynamics of tacrolimus in solid organ transplantation. Clin Pharmacokin 2004;43(10):623–53.

33. Sarna S, Hoppu K, Neovonen PH, et al. Methylprednisolone exposure, rather than dose, predicts adrenal suppression and growth inhibition in children with liver and renal transplant. J Clin Endocrinol Metab 1997;82(1):75–7.

34. Kuypers DR. Influence of interactions between immunosuppressive drugs on therapeutic drug monitoring. Ann Transplant 2008;13:11–8.

35. Pescovitz MD, Conti D, Dunn J, et al. Intravenous mycophenolate mofetil: safety, tolerability, and pharmacokinetics. Clin Transplant 2000;14:179–88.

36. Kuypers DRJ. Immunosuppressive drug monitoring—what to use in clinical practice today to improve renal graft outcome. Transplant Internatl 2005;18:140–50.

37. Cox MC, Ensom MHH. Mycophenolate mofetil for solid organ transplantation: does the evidence support the need for clinical pharmacokinetic monitoring? Ther Drug Monit 2003;23:534–42.

38. Lancaster DL, Patel N, Lennard L, et al. 6-Thioguanine in children with acute lymphoblastic leukemia: influence of food on parent drug pharmacokinetics and 6-thioguanine nucleotide concentrations. Br J Clin Pharmacol 2001;51:531–9.

39. Gearry RB, Day AS, Barclay ML, et al. Azathioprine and allopurinol: a two-edged interaction. J Gastroenterol Hepatol 2010;25(4):653–5.

40. Kahan BD, Camardo JS. Rapamycin: clinical results and future opportunities. Transplantation 2001;72:1181.

41. Saunders RN, Metcalfe MS, Nicholson ML. Rapamycin in transplantation: a review of the evidence. Kidney Int 2001;59(1):3–16.

42. Kahan BD, Napoli KL, Kelly PA, et al. Therapeutic monitoring of sirolimus: correlations with efficacy and toxicity. Clin Transplant 2000;14:97–109.

43. Chueh SCJ, Kahan BD. Dyslipidemia in renal transplant recipients treated with a sirolimus and cyclosporine-based immunosuppressive regimen: incidence, risk factors, progression, and prognosis. Transplantation 2003;76:375–82.

44. Stallone G, Infante B, Grandaliano G, et al. Management of side effects of sirolimus therapy. Transplantation 2009;87(8 Suppl):S23–6.

45. Guibeau JM. Delayed wound healing with sirolimus after liver transplant. Am J Pharmacother 2002;36:1391–5.

46. van Gelder T, ter Meulen CG, Hené R, et al. Oral ulcers in kidney transplant recipients treated with sirolimus and mycophenolate mofetil. Transplantation 2003;75:788–91.

47. Pallet N, Thervet E, Legendre C, et al. Sirolimus early graft nephrotoxicity: clinical and experimental data. Curr Drug Safety 2006;1(2):179–87.

48. Zortress® (everolimus) Product Information. Novartis Pharmaceuticals Corporation, East Hanover, NJ, 2010.
49. Oellerich M, Hon, Armstrong VW. The role of therapeutic drug monitoring in individualizing immunosuppressive drug therapy: recent developments. Ther Drug Monit 2006;28:720–5.
50. Emamaullee J, Toso C, Merani S, et al. Costimulatory blockade with belatacept in clinical and experimental transplantation—a review. Expert Opin Biol Ther 2009;9(6):789–96.
51. Vincenti F. Costimulation blockade in autoimmunity and transplantation. J Allergy Clin Immunol 2008;121(2);299–306.
52. Vincenti F, Larsen C, Durrbach A, et al. Costimulation blockade with belatacept in renal transplantation. New Engl J Med 2005;353(8):770–81.
53. Brennan CD, Flavin K, Lowell JA, et al. A randomized, double-blinded comparison of Thymoglobulin versus Atgam for induction immunosuppressive therapy in adult renal transplant recipients. Transplantation 1999;67(7):1011–8.
54. Marvin MR, Drogan C, Sawinski D, et al. Administration of rabbit antithymocyte globulin (Thymoglobulin) in ambulatory renal-transplant patients. Transplantation 2003;75(4):488–9.
55. Bloom DD, Hu H, Fechner JH, et al. T-lymphocyte alloresponses of Campath-1H-treated kidney transplant patients. Transplantation 2006;81(1):81–7.
56. Tan HP, Smaldone MD, Shapiro R. Immunosuppressive preconditioning or induction regimens: evidence to date. Drugs 2006;66:1535–45.
57. Bush WW. Overview of transplantation immunology and the pharmacotherapy of adult solid organ transplant recipients: focus on immunosuppression. AACN Clin Issues 1999;10(2):253–69.
58. Kovarik J, Breidenbach T, Berveau C, et al. Disposition and immunodynamics of basiliximab in liver allograft recipients. Clin Pharmacol Ther 1998;64:66–72.
59. Everly JJ, Walsh RC, Alloway RR, et al. Proteosome inhibition for antibody-mediated rejection. Curr Opin Organ Transplant 2009;14:662–6.
60. Parker A, Bowles K, Bradley JA, et al. Management of post-transplant lymphoproliferative disorder in adult solid organ transplant recipients—BCSH and BTS Guidelines. Br J Haematol 2010;149(5):693–705.
61. Kaposztas Z, Podder H, Mauiyyedi S, et al. Impact of rituximab therapy for treatment of acute humoral rejection. Clin Transplant 2009;23(1):63–73.
62. Vo A, Peng A, Toyoda M, et al. Use of intravenous immune globulin and rituximab for desensitization of highly HLA-sensitized patients awaiting kidney transplantation. Transplantation 2010;89(9):1095–102.

Nursing Care of the Pancreas Transplant Recipient

Michelle M. James, MS, RN, CNS, CCTN

KEYWORDS

- Diabetes mellitus • Immunosuppression • Nursing care
- Pancreas transplantation

Pancreas transplantation was first successfully performed (simultaneously with a kidney transplant) at the University of Minnesota in Minneapolis in 1966 by Drs Richard Lillehei and William Kelly.[1,2] The first two recipients achieved the goal of insulin independence, albeit for short time spans of only months, but were plagued by complications. The first simultaneous kidney and pancreas grafts failed because of pancreatic fistula and rejection,[1,3] but the patient ultimately died of pulmonary embolism, and the second recipient died 5 months posttransplant with functioning grafts of infection after experiencing multiple rejection episodes.[2,4] However, these two cases demonstrated that euglycemia could be restored with a pancreas transplant graft, forever altering the future of transplantation. Although slow to gain broad acceptance, pancreas transplants became widely performed with the introduction of cyclosporine to the transplant community in 1983,[5] resulting in more than 30,000 pancreas transplants performed as of December 31, 2008, according to the International Pancreas Transplant Registry (IPTR).[6]

POTENTIAL COMPLICATIONS OF HYPOGLYCEMIA AND HYPERGLYCEMIA

Virtually all pancreas transplants (96.6% according to IPTR)[6] are performed for the purpose of achieving a euglycemic state in a patient with c-peptide–deficient insulin-dependent diabetes mellitus (DM).[5,7] C-peptide deficient diabetes is most often type 1 diabetes. Type 1 DM, which includes only 5% to 10% of all persons who have diabetes, results from autoimmune destruction of pancreatic beta cells (Ohler, p 557).[8] Beta cells of the islets of Langerhans are the endocrine cells of the pancreas that produce insulin. Type 2 DM, which affects 90% to 95% of persons who have diabetes and is the type currently rising rapidly in children and adolescents, is differentiated from type 1 as production of insulin by the beta cells but presence of insulin resistance leading to deficiency.[8] In both type 1 and type 2 DM the exocrine

Department of Nursing, University of Minnesota Medical Center, Fairview, Minneapolis, MN, USA
E-mail address: MJAMES2@Fairview.org

Crit Care Nurs Clin N Am 23 (2011) 425–441
doi:10.1016/j.ccell.2011.07.001
0899-5885/11/$ – see front matter © 2011 Elsevier Inc. All rights reserved.

function of the pancreas, secretion of amylase and lipase into the intestine to assist with the breakdown of food, is unaffected.

Euglycemia is an important achievement because the consequences of the insufficient insulin secretion by the beta cells of the pancreas in DM cause significant complications. According to the Diabetes Control and Complications Trial, glycosylated hemoglobin levels decreased to near normal state by intensive insulin therapy significantly reduced the rate of secondary complications in the patient with diabetes. Total elimination of secondary complications could only be achieved by "perfect" control, a formidable challenge even with today's technologically sophisticated glucose monitoring and insulin delivery devices.[5,7] In light of the evidence that perfect control best addresses, or prevents, secondary complications of insulin insufficiency caused by diabetes, the achievement of euglycemia with pancreas transplantation is a logical choice.

Hyperglycemia and hypoglycemia both cause considerable morbidity and play a strong role in mortality. In hyperglycemia, excess glucose collects in or along the walls of vessels. With increasing duration and severity of hyperglycemia, specific microvascular, macrovascular, and neurologic complications (also called diabetic triopathy) can develop and worsen.

Microvascular complications include retinopathy and nephropathy. Diabetic nephropathy originates with glucose attachment to the walls of the glomeruli of the kidney, leading to thick, sclerosed vessels through which blood flow is impeded.[9] Hyperglycemia also causes glycosuria, which triggers reabsorption of glucose attached to sodium, resulting in high systemic sodium levels and as such, fluid volume excess. The heart then reacts to fluid volume overload by releasing atrial natriuretic peptide to promote diuresis. However, this dieresis increases intraglomerular pressure, thus causing more damage and glomerulosclerosis.[10] Concurrently, glomeruli allow protein, specifically albumin, to spill into the urine. Ultimately, the combination results in kidney failure.[10] Seventy-three percent of adults with DM have hypertension, and diabetic nephropathy is the leading cause of kidney failure in the United States.[7]

Retinopathy occurs when collection of excess glucose in the retinal vessels results in ischemia, which in turn promotes growth of new, tenuous vessels near the optic nerve that rupture easily. In the presence of hypertension, hemorrhage, fibrosis, and retinal detachment can occur, culminating in partial or full blindness. Diabetic retinopathy is the leading cause of new cases of blindness in adults aged 20 to 74 in the United States.[11]

Macrovascular complications of diabetes include such dangerous clinical conditions as cerebrovascular accident (CVA), myocardial infarction (MI), and peripheral arterial disease (PAD). The occurrence of macrovascular events correlates directly with hemoglobin A1c levels—the higher the level, the greater risk of such an event or complication. In the setting of hyperglycemia, glucose attachment to the walls of blood vessels causes stiffening and sclerosis of the vessel walls, which can lead to tears in the walls. In the presence of dyslipidemia, the tears in the walls allow plaque to leak into the vessel, causing a macrovascular event like a CVA or MI. More concerning, CVAs and MI death rates are 2 to 4 times higher in persons who have diabetes than in adults who do not.[11] This increase is thought to correlate with the absence of chest pain in 50% of persons who have diabetes; if chest pain is not perceived, treatment will not be sought, and care is at minimum dangerously delayed. In the case of PAD, repeated events cause blockage of vessels to the extremities, necessitating amputation. More than 60% of nontraumatic amputations occur in persons who have diabetes.[11]

Neuropathic complications also arise in the presence of diabetic hyperglycemia. Excess glucose damages the nerve structure and decreases blood flow to the nerves. The damage to the nerve can cause inaccurate perception, numbness, tingling, and allodynia (pain that is inappropriately severe given the stimuli for pain). Later, the nerve dies, and sensation ceases.[12] Different kinds of neuropathy can occur in persons who have diabetes. The most commonly discussed is peripheral neuropathy. Peripheral neuropathy, which occurs primarily in the extremities of the body, commonly causes numbness, tingling, and allodynia.[10] For example, a patient experiencing peripheral neuropathy describes extreme foot pain (because the sural nerve, one of the longest of the body, is the usually the first afflicted in diabetic neuropathic pain) when a sheet is placed gently over the lower extremities. Later, the same person who experienced allodynia of the foot loses perception in the foot, and gait is therefore impaired because it is difficult to ambulate when unable to perceive the foot touching the floor. This inability to perceive the foot results in a flat-footed, stomping type of gait instead of the usual heel-to-toe gait.

Less often discussed is the second form of neuropathy some persons who have diabetes experience, autonomic neuropathy. These neuropathies affect organ systems of the body, altering function. Development of neuropathies directly correlates with progression of diabetes and glycemic control.[10] Orthostatic hypotension, the body's inability to compensate for postural alteration resulting in decreased cerebral perfusion, is a consequence of autonomic neuropathy of the cardiovascular system. Gastroparesis is also a form of autonomic neuropathy found in persons who have advanced diabetes. Because of glucose collection within the small vessels and nerves of the intestine, gastrointestinal (GI) system dysfunction occurs. Gastroparesis involves delayed and often dysfunctional gastric emptying, resulting in both constipation and diarrhea. The genitourinary system can also be affected by autonomic neuropathy, commonly a neurogenic bladder. In this form of diabetic neuropathy, the ability to sense a full bladder and as such drain it properly is lost. This loss of sensation results in higher postvoid residuals and decreased voiding and development of urinary tract infections.

Finally, autonomic neuropathy and insulin production deficiency may reduce counter-regulatory hormone release, preventing the body from generating its own glucose or the ability to sense hypoglycemia, called *hypoglycemic unawareness*. When the person who has diabetes is unaware that glucose levels are low or dropping, there is no awareness of the need to compensate by consuming carbohydrates. This unawareness can result in dangerously low glucose levels and potentially death.[10]

PANCREAS TRANSPLANTATION OPTIONS

As stated earlier, pancreas transplantation is indicated in diabetes, most often specifically advanced type 1 diabetes, in which the pancreas produces little or no insulin. The hope is to restore endocrine function and a euglycemic state.[5] However, transplantation requires immunosuppression to prevent rejection of the new graft. With immunosuppression come other potential side effects including but not limited to nephrotoxicity and higher infection and malignancy risks.[8] Other potential risks that accompany all large surgical procedures (ie. MI, deep vein thrombosis, pulmonary embolism)[8] are also possible in the pancreas transplant surgery and may pose a higher risk because of the complications of diabetes.[5]

In weighing the risks with pancreas transplantation described previously, the benefits of euglycemia provided by pancreas transplantation are generally considered to outweigh the risks of immunosuppression in two situations: patients with end-stage renal disease secondary to diabetic nephropathy or when the patient already requires immunosuppression for a previous kidney transplant.[5,13] In the first situation, in which the patient is essentially experiencing failure of both native kidney and pancreas organs, a simultaneous pancreas and kidney (SPK) is indicated. SPKs are the most common method of pancreas transplantation, constituting 72% of all pancreas transplants performed in the United States.[6] The biggest advantages to SPK include that both uremia and diabetes are addressed in one surgery[5] and there are higher long-term graft survival rates than those of pancreas after kidney (PAK) transplant or pancreas transplant alone (PTA).

However, the wait time on the deceased donor list for SPK is the longest of the pancreas transplants,[6] primarily because of the high need for deceased donor kidney transplants.[5,7] To prevent the long wait on the deceased donor list and yet reap the advantages of receiving both the kidney and pancreas grafts in one surgery, a simultaneous living donor kidney transplant and deceased donor pancreas transplant could also be considered. In this situation, an appropriately matched living donor kidney recipient joins the potential recipient in traveling to the hospital to donate his/her kidney at the same time a suitable deceased donor pancreas becomes available, resulting in one surgery wherein both the living donor kidney and deceased donor pancreas are simultaneously transplanted.[5] This recipient then benefits from both the statistically significant longevity of a living donor kidney (vs a deceased donor kidney transplant),[7] as well as the shorter wait time for the separate PTA deceased donor list[6] before achieving insulin independence with a functioning pancreas graft. Coordination of this transplant event can be challenging[7] because two operating rooms are necessary at whatever hour the pancreas is ready to be transplanted into the recipient. Furthermore, medical providers and nurses caring for patients with the simultaneous living donor kidney/deceased donor pancreas must be aware that while transplanted at the same time, each organ is from a different donor and as such, the immunologic profile and resulting rejection potential differs between the organs. Thus, both organs must be monitored separately for rejection.[7]

The second most common situation in which the benefits of euglycemia provided by pancreas transplantation are generally considered to outweigh the risks of immunosuppression transplant is when a kidney transplant is already present, occurring in 21% of pancreas transplants.[6] In this case, a PAK transplant is appropriate because the risks of immunosuppression are already assumed by the patient for the kidney transplant, and as such only surgical complications are the potential risks in a PAK surgery.[5] Whereas this situation obviously involves two surgeries to achieve the same results as one SPK surgery, both surgeries are smaller procedures with less extensive dissection and seem to be better tolerated.[5,7] As stated earlier, waiting time on the deceased donor list is also shortest for the pancreas alone,[6] an important factor to consider in light of the progression of diabetic complications during the wait for an organ. Equally noteworthy in this situation, as well as the earlier described simultaneous living donor kidney/deceased donor pancreas, is that a living donor kidney may be used, avoiding the use of the corresponding deceased donor kidney and thereby expanding the deceased donor kidney pool.

The final and least common situation in which the benefits of euglycemia can be provided by pancreas transplantation is PTA. PTA accounts for only 8% of total pancreas transplants.[6] A PTA is potential solution for the nonuremic person with diabetes who has such severe hypoglycemic unawareness that it is a significant safety or quality of life issue for the potential recipient.[5,7] Of all the pancreas transplant strategies, PTA draws the most criticism because immunosuppression is not required for another organ, only for the pancreas itself. Thus the argument for trading insulin injections for immunosuppressive complications is most vehement in this strategy.[1,5,13,14] It must, however, be considered that pancreas transplantation can solely stabilize or improve the secondary complications of diabetes including diabetic nephropathy,[5,7] potentially avoiding the need for future kidney transplantation if performed in the early stages of nephropathy and providing improved quality of life in a newly euglycemic state.[5,7,15]

INDICATIONS AND CONTRAINDICATIONS FOR PANCREAS TRANSPLANTATION

The main indication for pancreas transplant, as stated earlier, is type 1 DM. However, because three strategies for pancreas transplantation exist, further clarification of the ideal option can be articulated. A person who has uremic type 1 diabetes should always be considered for a SPK, ideally preemptive to dialysis,[1,5] or a PAK. The American Diabetes Association also recommends that indications for pancreas transplant include "history of frequent, acute, and severe metabolic complications (eg, hypoglycemia, hyperglycemia, ketoacidosis), incapacitating clinical and emotional problems with exogenous insulin prescription, and consistent failure of insulin-based management to prevent acute complications."[5] Insulin independent persons who have diabetes without uremia who suffer with severe hypoglycemic unawareness or worsening secondary complications of diabetes should also be considered for a PTA.[5]

Contraindications to pancreas transplant are similar among potential recipients of all organs.[1,5,7] These contraindications include recent malignancy, active infections, noncompliance, liver cirrhosis, and serious psychiatric or psychosocial illness. However, extra focus should be placed on those complications common to diabetes. Unaddressed cardiovascular disease is a significant contraindication in pancreas transplantation[5,7] because one of the major complications of diabetes is coronary artery disease. Even young persons with type 1 diabetes may have severe coronary artery disease, posing greater operative and postoperative mortality risks.[1] Advanced vascular disease, common in persons with diabetes, also poses significant operative risk and should be thoroughly evaluated.[5,7] Iliac artery stenosis specifically is an important risk factor for pancreas transplantation, because anastomosis to the iliac artery is required in the operative procedure.[5]

EVALUATION FOR PANCREAS TRANSPLANTATION

Assessment of appropriate candidacy for pancreas transplantation is designed to verify ability to tolerate the surgical risk of the transplantation as well as the potential risks inherent to chronic immunosuppression. Evaluation can be simplified into a few important categories: infection risk/status, cancer risk/status, general health and candidacy status, social and financial health status, immunogenetics, and, with a greater focus in pancreas transplantation, cardiac and vascular health status.

Infection and cancer risk are important to evaluate in all transplant candidates because immunosuppression lessens the body's ability to find and fight infection or cancer cells. Tests commonly performed for infection and cancer include chest radiograph, urinalysis, prostate-specific antigen in men and Pap smear and mammogram in women, and sigmoidoscopy or colonoscopy.[8] Serologies for cytomegalovirus, human immunodeficiency virus, and Epstein-Barr virus are also performed. None of the aforementioned serologies are contraindications for pancreas transplantation, but pretransplant status is important to know for baseline comparison purposes because each is necessary to be monitored for potential complications posttransplant.

The sigmoidoscopy or colonoscopy (and perhaps further GI evaluation if indicated) can also provide valuable information regarding autonomic dysfunction, commonly manifested as gastroparesis in the patient who has diabetes. The status of the potential recipient's gastroparesis is helpful in preparation for posttransplant recovery because anesthesia commonly temporarily worsens it,[16] as may some of the immunosuppressant medications.[5]

General health and candidacy status indicate the potential transplant recipient's current health as well as need for pancreas transplant. Electrolyte panel, phosphorus and magnesium levels, complete blood count with differential, and thyroid function studies are commonly performed for this purpose. Liver function and liver disease are also assessed by performing liver function tests; hepatitis A immunoglobulin, hepatitis B (surface antigen, antibody, and core antigen) and hepatitis C (antibody) serologies; and if indicated, liver biopsy, to rule out hepatic insufficiency and viral hepatitis. These assessments are performed because the presence of hepatitis B or C has been associated with worse long-term outcomes in nonhepatic transplants.[5]

Kidney function is also assessed to either indicate need for SPK or validate that kidney transplantation is unnecessary in potential PTA recipients. Along with the creatinine in the electrolyte panel, kidney function is measured by glomerular filtration rate, blood urea nitrogen (BUN) level, and 24-hour protein/creatinine clearance test. Bone density scan may also be performed, especially if the potential recipient is expected to take prednisone long-term posttransplant per the transplant center's protocol because it impacts bone density. The status of the native pancreas is assessed via C peptide (a byproduct of insulin production), hemoglobin A1c, and amylase and lipase blood serum levels.[8] Last, if bladder drainage is anticipated, urologic examination including, for example, a voiding cystourethrogram is recommended to ensure proper drainage of urine from the bladder. Dysfunctional drainage of pancreatic exocrine products in bladder-drained pancreas transplants predisposes the recipient to graft pancreatitis.[5]

Social and financial health status requires evaluation because of their central role in maintenance of the pancreas graft. Psychosocial evaluation includes assessment of the transplant candidate's psychological health and potential social support postoperatively to ensure assistance in coping with the significant new requirements of maintaining the transplanted pancreas. Lack of adequate support may impact health maintenance posttransplant. Financial assessment is also important, especially related to insurance coverage versus patient responsibilities. Costs of medications alone can be immense, and as such assessment of the candidate's ability to pay for his/her portion of the cost must be addressed to ensure that noncompliance with the medications due entirely to lack of ability to pay for them is avoided if at all possible.[16]

Immunologic assessment is essential in all transplant recipients to ensure proper matching of grafted organs with potential recipients, thereby preventing rejection of the new organ. ABO compatibility is crucial in pancreas transplant, thus blood typing is performed. Panel-reactive antibody and human leukocyte antigen (HLA) typing are also performed. However, it is generally accepted that HLA matching is not associated with graft outcomes in SPK recipients and is potentially unimportant for PAK and PTA graft outcomes,[5] resulting in 56% of SPK recipients and 37% of PTA recipients receiving HLA mismatch grafts according to the IPTR.[6]

Cardiac and vascular health status requires a more in-depth focus when assessing a pancreas transplant candidate because of cardiovascular comorbidities with diabetes. Therefore, not only are a fasting lipid panel and coagulation profile indicated, but also a 12-lead electrocardiogram (EKG) and echocardiogram, as well as cardiologic clearance that may include any of the following tests: carotid artery, femoral, or peripheral vessels ultrasounds; dobutamine stress echocardiogram; nuclear stress test; cardiac catheterization; and coronary angiogram.[5,8]

If the patient is deemed safe to undergo the pancreas transplant, she/he will be listed on the United Network of Organ Sharing list. As stated earlier, the PTA and SPK lists are separate, so the patient, with the help and education of the interdisciplinary team, must decide on which to be listed. When an appropriately matched organ is found, the patient is called in for transplant. At that time, laboratory tests including complete blood cell count, electrolyte levels, Immunologic crossmatch, infectious disease antibodies levels, as well as chest radiographs, and EKG are repeated to verify the patient is currently safe to undergo transplantation.[8] Induction immunosuppression may be administered preoperatively or intraoperatively based on the protocol of the transplant program.[8] Patients often require emotional support in the immediate preoperative time frame. Excitement and anxiety are commonly expressed at this time.[8]

PANCREAS TRANSPLANT SURGERY

Two surgical methods of pancreas transplantation are possible to achieve the three transplantation scenarios described earlier (SPK, PAK, and PTA): solitary pancreas transplant is used for PAK and PTA as opposed to the SPK surgery, which is similar to the PTA but more extensive because of the kidney transplant immediately after pancreas transplantation.[3] In the SPK transplant, the kidney is transplanted after the pancreas transplant, usually on the contralateral iliac fossa either intraperitoneally or extraperitoneally.[3]

Upon arrival, the donor pancreas includes the entire pancreas, a duodenal segment, and its attached arterial and venous blood vessels. Midline incision (vs iliac or transverse abdominal incision options) is preferred to enter the abdomen because it reduces the incidence of wound infections and is easier to place organs,[3] but may also decrease GI motility.[16] The denervated pancreas graft is usually heterotopically placed intraperitoneally on the right side of the pelvis.[7] The native pancreas is not removed. This placement provides easier access to the right iliac vessels,[3] lower rate of allograft thrombosis, easier access for percutaneous biopsy, and the option to choose bladder or enteric drainage of the exocrine secretions of the pancreas graft.[7]

Determination of the best method for pancreatic exocrine secretions via bladder or enteric drainage remains a debated topic among surgeons because of the positive and negative aspects inherent to both methods. Bladder drainage had been favored in the 1980s and 1990s by transplant surgeons for exocrine drainage but is now used in only 10% to 20% of pancreas transplants.[6] Bladder-drained pancreas transplantation involves a side-to-side anastomosis between the duodenum segment attached to the donor pancreas and the recipient's bladder (**Fig. 1**).[7] The major advantage to bladder drainage is that exocrine products, specifically amylase, in the urine provide a noninvasive direct marker for graft function. When collected and analyzed, lower levels of urine amylase provide an early and sensitive, although not terribly specific, indication of acute pancreas rejection.[5] In addition, this pancreas placement also allows for easier biopsy[17] because the pancreas is not "wrapped up" in intestine, a possibility in enteric drainage that could lead to unintentional perforation of the intestine during an attempted pancreas biopsy. As such, rejection is detected early with bladder-drained pancreas transplants, resulting in lower rejection loss rates than with enteric drainage.[5] Bladder drainage also avoids exacerbation of gastroparesis and contamination of the graft with enteric contents, both of which can occur with enteric drainage.[7] However, the large quantities of bicarbonate (<2 L/d[16]) also produced by the pancreas, normally reabsorbed into the large intestine, are incorporated into the

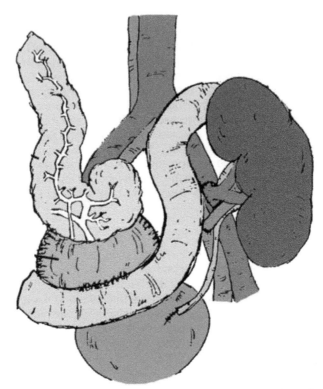

Fig. 1. Surgical techniques in simultaneous pancreas-kidney transplantation. (*A*) Enteric drainage of pancreatic exocrine secretions. (*B*) Bladder drainage of pancreatic exocrine secretions. (*Adapted from* Steen,79 copyright 1999, with permission from Lippincott Williams & Wilkins/American Association of Critical-Care Nurses.)

urine and drained out of the body. Depletion of this metabolic base can lead to dehydration, hypovolemia, and metabolic (specifically hyperchloremic) acidosis if uncorrected.[1,3,7,8] The presence of bicarbonate also decreases the acidity of the urine, predisposing the bladder-drained pancreas recipient to urinary tract infections.[3,17] Other urologic complications with this method include urethritis, hematuria, and urinary reflux into the pancreas graft causing pancreatitis.[3,5,7] If any of the aforementioned complications become significant, enteric conversion, in which the exocrine drainage is surgically altered to drain into the intestine instead of the bladder, is an option. Enteric conversion is not usually performed until 6 to 12 months posttransplant to allow for postoperative recovery, but also because the immunologic monitoring advantage of bladder drainage decreases after that time because of lower rejection rates.[3,5] Approximately 10% to 25% of bladder-drained pancreas transplant recipients are converted to enteric drainage by 5 years posttransplant.[3,7,8]

The earliest favored method of drainage was most similar to natural anatomy, enteric drainage. Enteric drainage fell out of favor because of intraabdominal abscesses from anastomotic leaks in the early years of pancreas transplantation. This method is, again the favored method of exocrine drainage because of improvements in surgical techniques[6,18] resulting in infection rates comparable to bladder-drained pancreas transplant recipients.[6] In enteric drainage, the donor duodenum and attached pancreas are anastomosed to the recipients jejunum for purposes of draining the pancreatic exocrine products into the GI system (see **Fig. 1**). The positive aspects of enteric drainage include avoidance of urinary tract infections and other urologic complications, decreased risk of dehydration and electrolyte abnormalities,[7,5] and lower graft pancreatitis rates.[6] Enteric drainage is often chosen in SPK recipients because pancreas rejection can be monitored by creatinine levels, because the immunologic profile for the kidney and pancreas are the same.[5,8] In that situation, the immunologic advantage to bladder drainage is unnecessary, and avoidance of urologic complications with enteric drainage is ideal.[5,8] However, whereas rates of infection, anastomotic leaks, and bleeding are similar between bladder and enteric drainage, the technical failure rate is higher in enteric-drained pancreas transplantation.[6]

Before surgical incision, broad-spectrum antibiotics and antifungals are commonly infused to prevent infection during surgery and immediately postoperatively.[5] During the pancreas transplant surgical procedure, maintenance of normalized glucose levels with continuous intravenous (IV) insulin infusion is essential.[5] In all three categories of pancreas transplantation (SPK, PTA, and PAK) most recipients receive depleting antibody medications, potentially in combination with nondepleting antibodies.[6] Although debatable among transplant clinicians, many centers also use some form of prophylactic anticoagulation to prevent pancreas graft thrombosis during surgery and/or postoperatively. Methods and results of thrombosis prevention among centers vary.[5,8,19]

ISLET CELL REPLACEMENT

Although currently still in clinical research, islet cell replacement is an option to restore euglycemia in a patient with diabetes. In islet cell replacement, the deceased donor pancreas is enzymatically and physically degraded, and the insulin-producing cells, islets of Langerhans, or simply islets, are removed. The islet cells are then infused into the recipient. Whereas the concept of islet transplantation has existed since the early days of pancreas transplantation, long-term insulin independence has remained a challenge, and as such it has been performed only in clinical trials. The Edmonton protocol from the University of Alberta, Canada, rejuvenated interest in islet transplantation when it was reported in 2000 that all 7 trial patients remained free of insulin at 1 year post–islet infusion using a prednisone-free immunosuppressant protocol.[5] However, at 5 years, only 10% of the islet recipients were insulin independent, and a multicenter trial did not replicate such results.[5] Instead, only 53% of patients were reported to be free of insulin at 1 year.[13] Thus, clinical trials continue in the hope of achieving surgery-free long-term insulin independence.

POSTOPERATIVE NURSING CARE

After surgery the pancreas transplant recipient recovers in the postanesthesia care unit. Thereafter the patient may be transferred to the intensive care unit or to a transplant or specialized monitoring unit, because cardiac monitoring is common for 24 to 48 hours post–pancreas transplant, especially if the patient had a preexisting cardiac history.[8] Similar to all surgical patients, hemodynamic stability, fluid and electrolyte balance, and adequate cardiorespiratory function must be frequently assessed and maintained during the immediate postoperative period.[5] This assessment includes vital signs, central venous pressure (CVP) monitoring, intake/output measurement and potentially replacement, oxygen saturation monitoring, laboratory value trend monitoring, and correlation of the aforementioned data with the head-to-toe nursing assessment to diagnose, intervene, and potentially prevent complications.[8]

Some components of postoperative monitoring and assessment are unique to the pancreas transplant recipient. Whereas the impact of inappropriate fluid and electrolyte balance can have significant consequences like fluid overload and dehydration in other surgical patients, intravascular volume must be maintained in the pancreas transplant recipient because the pancreas is a low-flow organ.[5] The grafted pancreas requires adequate perfusion to prevent thrombosis of the graft, which is most likely to occur within 24 to 48 hours posttransplant.[8] As such, CVP, urine output, and heart rate and blood pressure monitoring in conjunction with correlation of laboratory values indicating dehydration (decreased hemoglobin, increased hematocrit, increased BUN or creatinine) are paramount to this population. Each transplant center has its own protocol for maintenance of appropriate hydration. The protocols may include continuous administration of maintenance IV fluids or replacement of nasogastric (NG) and urine output, in conjunction with IV fluid boluses as needed.[8] Commonly, programs also have a separate protocol for frequency of urine assessment and replacement for the SPK transplant recipient.

Fluid management is more challenging in the bladder-drained pancreas transplant recipient, both immediately postoperatively as well as postdischarge, because of the loss of potentially 2 L of fluid exocrine secretions through the bladder.[8,16] Recognizing that the loss of the exocrine product bicarbonate may lead to orthostatic hypotension, metabolic acidosis, or potentiate dehydration, IV fluids often contain bicarbonate, and oral supplementation is initiated after the diet is advanced.[8,16] Patients experiencing orthostatic hypotension need to be taught rise slowly from a lying position and sit for a moment before standing to prevent falls.[16] They also need to be taught to drink enough fluids to remain adequately hydrated upon discharge, a bigger challenge for SPK recipients who were on fluid restrictions because of dialysis pretransplant.[8,16] It is not uncommon for bladder-drained pancreas recipients to require IV fluid boluses postdischarge, but it is generally limited to the first 3 months posttransplant.[16]

Beyond hydration, monitoring proper functioning of the new pancreas is of the utmost importance. Elevated serum laboratory levels of amylase and lipase, produced by the alpha cells of the pancreas, are generally considered the first sign of rejection.[5,7,8] However, these levels may be temporarily elevated for 48 to 96 hours posttransplant in a mild form of pancreatitis due to cold ischemia injury and handling in surgery. Therefore, early posttransplant elevation of serum amylase and lipase may be inaccurate predictors of rejection at that time.[8] In the SPK recipient, creatinine is also closely monitored posttransplant with the assumption that the high levels before surgery will immediately decrease postoperatively. If, however, creatinine levels rise postoperatively, it can be a sign of dehydration or rejection of the kidney. In that the kidney and pancreas are immunologically identical in the SPK recipient, increased creatinine level is a biomarker for pancreas rejection as well.[5,7] Urine amylase secretion can also be collected and analyzed in bladder-drained pancreas transplant recipients as a noninvasive method to monitor for rejection.[5,8] This analysis is usually conducted by collecting all urine for an 8-hour period daily during the posttransplant stay. The urine is then analyzed for hourly average contents. The hourly average can then be compared with a different day's contents, and an unexplained decrease in the level of urine amylase is a sign of rejection.[8]

Blood glucose levels are monitored posttransplant as well, often hourly or every other hour, especially in the presence of an insulin infusion.[8] Insulin infusions are used in many centers postoperatively to maintain tight glucose control and "rest" the insulin-producing cells of the pancreas,[5] because hyperglycemia may occur as a side effect of high-dose corticosteroids.[8] Sudden unexplained sharp rise in glucose level and/or amylase and lipase levels is indicative of pancreas thrombosis.[5,8] If this rise occurs, the medical team should be immediately contacted with the anticipation of an emergent ultrasound to assess patency of blood flow to the graft.[5] If thrombosis is discovered, potential emergent reoperation is anticipated in the hope of salvaging the graft.[8]

An NG tube, a central intravenous catheter, surgical or pancreatic drains, and a urinary catheter are also be placed intraoperatively, and all remain intact postoperatively.[8,16] The NG tube is placed to address surgically induced decreased GI function, a potentially significant issue if diabetic gastroparesis was present before surgery.[16] The NG tube usually remains for 1 to 2 days postoperatively to suction gastric contents, but potentially longer if nausea and vomiting persist or in the presence of a postoperative ileus.[8] The central IV catheter is important for infusion of parenteral medications and fluids, CVP measurement of intravascular volume status, and blood samples for laboratory analysis.[8] This catheter may remain for the duration of the hospitalization, depending on the needs of the patient and individual transplant center protocols. Surgical or pancreatic drains may be placed in the operating room to monitor anastomotic leaks or other surgical complications. These drains should be measured and assessed often for changes in amount and appearance to determine potential internal issues at the site of the pancreas graft.[8] This assessment may include monitoring amylase levels of the drain contents as a sign of an anastomotic leak.[5,8] The urinary catheter placed in the operating room not only assists with the surgical procedure but also may be required to remain intact for days to weeks postoperatively in the case of the SPK or bladder-drained pancreas transplant, to allow healing of anastomoses to the bladder.

As stated earlier, immunosuppression, usually consisting of depleting antibody medications and potentially in combination with nondepleting antibodies, is initiated preoperatively or intraoperatively for pancreas transplant recipients.[5,6,8] Maintenance immunosuppression differs based on the protocol of the individual transplant program. Pancreas transplant protocols most often use tacrolimus and mycophenolate mofetil; however, a growing trend exists toward use of sirolimus, as monotherapy or in combination with other medications.[6] According to the IPTR, results were significantly better in centers with protocols using the aforementioned mediations.[6] Of note, steroid avoidance protocols are increasing in number with one-third of all SPK and PAK recipients receiving no initial or maintenance steroids.[6]

The length of stay in the hospital for the pancreas or SPK transplant recipient averages 7 to 14 days.[8] Whereas the patient is recovering physically from the surgery in the early part of the stay, emotional recovery is commonly part of the transplant experience as well.[8] The volume of new information, including activity restrictions, wound care, frequency of required physician and/or laboratory draw appointments, method of urine amylase collection, signs and symptoms of rejection and infection to look for and report to his/her coordinator, and many details about medications can be overwhelming. Education can ally concerns and prepare patients and families for how to best care for the new organs.[16] Patient education methods include individual education by pharmacists, coordinators, or staff nurses as well as classes, books, computer programs, and audiovisual materials.[16,20–24]

Knowledge of their medication regimen is extremely important for new transplant recipients. Reinforcement of the need to take immunosuppressant medications as directed for the entirety of the new organ's life span cannot be stressed enough, because the regimen is often complex.[8,20] Essential questions patients must be able to answer before discharge (and be repeated thereafter) are shown in **Box 1**.

SURGICAL COMPLICATIONS AFTER PANCREAS TRANSPLANTATION

Technical complication rate is higher in pancreas transplant recipients than after most other solid transplants.[14] The most concerning surgical complication is that of graft thrombosis, because it frequently results in pancreatectomy.[8,19,25] Pancreas thrombosis is statistically significantly higher (7%) in solitary pancreas transplant (PAK, PTA) when compared with SPK (5%).[6] Thrombosis also occurs more with enteric-drained pancreas transplants, but only statistically so in the SPK patient population.[6] Thrombosis occurs most frequently within 24 to 48 hours posttransplant and is usually venous in origin. Late thrombosis is possible, but is thought to be of immunologic origin.[19] Signs and symptoms of thrombosis include sudden, unexplained hyperglycemia, sharp rise in serum amylase or lipase levels, graft tenderness or enlargement, and in bladder-drained pancreas transplant recipients, massive hematuria and decrease in urine amylase.[8,5,18,25] Diagnosis is best confirmed with duplex Doppler ultrasound, contrast-enhanced computed tomography (CT) or magnetic resonance imaging, or relaparotomy.[18,25]

Most thromboses occur secondary to technical complications,[5,14,25] but in many pancreatectomy cases, no obvious technical "mistake" is present.[14] In the donor graft, a short portal vein, due to its requirement for extension grafting, and atherosclerotic vessels increase the risk of thrombosis.[5] Donor obesity, specifically body mass index greater than 30 kg/m^2, has been linked to increased risk of graft thrombosis.[14,19] Advanced donor age, cerebrovascular cause of death, organ preservation time greater than 24 hours, hemodynamic instability, and massive resuscitation are also considered risks of thrombosis.[7,14,18] In the recipient, atherosclerotic disease of the iliac artery, a technically difficult vascular anastomosis, and significant hematoma surrounding the vascular anastomosis can also lead to thrombosis.[5] Diabetes is actually a risk factor for thrombosis because it is a hypercoagulable state, as is hyperlipidemia, a common diabetic comorbidity, whereas coagulopathy related to uremia may offer some protection against thrombosis in SPK recipients.[7,18] In cases in which graft thrombosis occurred early posttransplant, especially in the first 2 to 4 weeks after surgery, pancreas retransplantation, possibly even concurrently with first allograft pancreatectomy, is possible with comparable results to first-time pancreas transplant.[19,25]

Another surgical complication is leakage through the anastomosis to the recipient. Implications of the pancreatic leak depend upon the method of exocrine drainage: bladder or enteric drainage. In the bladder-drained pancreas, the duodenum-bladder anastomosis allows urine to leak into the abdomen. Bladder leaks often occur soon (less than 4 wk) after transplant, but may occur later as well. Symptoms of leakage include abdominal pain, rise in serum amylase and lipase, and, potentially, fever.[7,8,18,25] Bladder-drained leaks are diagnosed via CT or cystoscopy and can usually by resolved nonsurgically by placement of a urinary catheter to drain the urine for 7 to 10 days.[5,18,25] If leakage does not resolve with urinary catheter drainage or is large upon presentation, enteric conversion may be warranted.[5,18,25] If severe infection occurs, patient mortality is the greater concern, and pancreatectomy may be appropriate.[18,25]

Enteric leaks were such a significant infectious concern in early pancreas transplant experience that bladder drainage became the favored method of exocrine drainage.[18,25] However, bladder drainage is again the favored method of exocrine drainage because improvements in surgical techniques have resulted in anastomotic leak rates similar to those of bladder-drained pancreas transplants.[6,18] In enteric drainage, leakage involves spillage of enteric contents into the abdomen and tends to cause early peritonitis and sepsis.[25] Early duodenal leaks tend to result from technical complications or increased preservation time, whereas late leaks tend to result from rejection, infection, or ischemia of the duodenal staple line.[7,14] Infections caused by enteric leaks tend to be fugal or gram-negative bacterial in origin, and may lead to pancreaticocutaneous fistula or peripancreatic abscess.[5,7] Symptoms are similar to intestinal perforation and include abdominal pain, fever, tachycardia, elevated white blood cells, elevated serum amylase, nausea and vomiting, and tenderness over graft site.[7,8,18,25] An enteric anastomotic leak usually requires relaparotomy, and based on severity of infection, potentially pancreatectomy.[5,7]

A third surgical complication of pancreas transplant, pancreatitis, is quite common, especially immediately postoperatively due to cold ischemia injury and handling in surgery.[7,8,18] Pancreatitis may produce temporary elevation of serum amylase and lipase levels for 48 to 96 hours posttransplant. Reflux pancreatitis in bladder-drained recipients may occur later posttransplant and involves urine flowing back into and irritating the grafted pancreas. This complication may occur as a result of incomplete bladder drainage, potentially due to preexisting neurogenic bladder concerns.[5] Symptoms include abdominal pain, graft tenderness, nausea and vomiting, ileus, and elevated serum amylase and lipase levels. It is important to rule out rejection when diagnosing pancreatitis, although abdominal pain is less likely in rejection.[8,18] Diagnosis and treatment of reflux pancreatitis requires insertion of a urinary catheter to drain the bladder. Recurrent reflux pancreatitis is an indication for enteric conversion.[25]

Late presentation of pancreatitis in an enteric-drained pancreas transplant is, however, more concerning and has unclear risk factors in origination.[25] CT is the best diagnostic method for pancreatitis, revealing a swollen, hypervascularized pancreas without a surrounding fluid collection.[18] Potential complications of pancreatitis include per-pancreatic abscess, pancreatic necrosis, or fistula.[25] Treatment includes conservative support of the pancreas; IV fluids, total parenteral nutrition instead of oral intake, antibiotics if deemed appropriate, and in some transplant centers, infusion of octreotide.[18,25] If the recipient deteriorates on this therapy or imaging suggests necrosis of part of the pancreas, relaparotomy may be required.[7,25]

Bleeding from pancreas anastomosis, resulting in either GI bleeding or hematuria, is also a postoperative concern for post–pancreas transplant recipients. This bleeding can be caused by ischemia/reperfusion injury of the donor duodenal segment attached to the pancreas or by a bleeding vessel at the suture line.[7] Discontinuation of anticoagulation should be considered in these situations. In the enteric-drained pancreas transplant recipient, this usually presents as lower GI bleeding. If it continues after discontinuation of anticoagulation, reexploration and evacuation of clots to prevent intraabdominal infection often results.[25] Hematuria in the bladder-drained recipient is not uncommon but usually resolves spontaneously and without significant patient or graft morbidity. If hematuria persists beyond discontinuation of anticoagulation, bladder irrigation and cystoscopy may be considered and generally produce successful outcomes with graft patency intact.[7,8] Although rare, hematuria can also be a sign of graft rejection or pancreas or kidney graft thrombosis.[8,25]

The surgical complication with the least likelihood of sequelae, cystitis, occurs in bladder-drained pancreas recipients only. The exocrine secretions are so corrosive to the urethra that it can be quite painful. Cystitis can be treated with insertion of a urinary catheter to allow healing, but frequent recurrence can be cause for enteric conversion.[8]

IMMUNOLOGIC COMPLICATIONS AFTER TRANSPLANT

Whereas fear of graft rejection causes recipients the most stress and worry,[16,26] improvements in immunosuppression have been responsible for remarkable decreases in immunologic graft losses.[14] One-year graft losses of immunologic origin are now 2% for SPK and 6% for both PAK and PTA recipients at 1 year posttransplant.[6] Moreover, the most frequent cause of graft loss in both PTA and PAK after 3 months is rejection, both acute and chronic types.[6] The rate of graft loss for all categories because of acute rejection peaks at 3 to 12 months and falls thereafter, whereas chronic graft loss rates steadily increase over time.[6] Enteric-drained versus bladder-drained pancreas transplants have similar outcomes in virtually every other aspect, but recipient category of enteric-drained PTA have higher immunologic graft loss rates.[5]

Early symptoms of acute (cellular) pancreas rejection are usually specific to injury to acinar cells, the originators of amylase and lipase, and include elevated serum amylase and/or lipase levels and significant decrease in urine amylase levels in the bladder-drained pancreas recipient.[5,7,8,27] In the SPK recipient, elevated creatinine signifies kidney rejection, which can be considered a surrogate marker for pancreas rejection as well.[7,27] The late symptom of pancreas rejection is hyperglycemia, when the beta cells of the islets of Langerhans become damaged, and usually signifies irreversible loss of the graft. Fever and tenderness over the graft are also potential signs of rejection.[5,7,8] However, pancreas rejection can only be diagnosed by ultrasound or CT-guided percutaneous needle biopsy of the pancreas.[5,7,8,27] Rejection confirmation requires immediate treatment with steroids and antilymphocyte therapy[5,8,17] and has a 90% reversal rate if diagnosed early.[17]

Unlike kidney transplantation, antibody-mediated rejection (AMR) of the pancreas has only recently been described in the literature.[27] Although AMR of the pancreas is poorly understood, it has been associated with hyperglycemia. Thus, unlike cellular rejection, it is theorized that injury to the beta cells occur in this pathology.[27] Diagnosis of pancreas AMR requirements are similar to kidney AMR: allograft dysfunction (increased serum amylase and/or lipase or hyperglycemia), a positive biopsy with the presence of C4d (a product of antibody-mediated immune response) but no chronic changes like fibrosis, and donor-specific antibody in serum.[7,27] Immediate and long-term effects of this diagnosis in pancreas transplant are not currently known.[27]

Chronic rejection can also occur in pancreas transplantation. Similar to other types of organ transplant, repeated acute pancreas rejection significantly increases the risk of graft loss due to chronic rejection.[27] Chronic rejection manifests as progressive need for insulin in pancreas recipients as a result of progressive fibrosis within the graft.[7] The level of cellular changes in chronic rejection has been shown to correlate with suboptimal immunosuppression; therefore, optimization is recommended to prevent progression of chronic rejection when suspected or detected in the grafted pancreas.[27]

OUTCOMES IN PANCREAS TRANSPLANTATION

According to the IPTR, 1-year and 3-year patient survival rates in all pancreas transplant categories (SPK, PAK, and PTA) have steadily improved. Rates now exceed 95% at 1 year and 90% at 3 years posttransplant in more than 22,000 pancreas transplants performed in the United States through the year-end of 2008. Pancreas 1-year graft function rates, however, differ due to immunologic graft loss among the categories: SPK was statistically significantly higher than PTA or PAK at 84.9%, 78.6%, and 78.9%, respectively.[6] This difference is even more noteworthy at 3 years posttransplant when immunologic graft loss between pancreas transplants between 2004 and 2008 was at 5% for SPK but nearly 15% for PAK, and almost 20% for PTA.

Most studies have also supported survival (graft and patient) benefit superior in pancreas recipients in comparison with deceased donor kidney recipients.[28] The value of solitary pancreas transplant, PAK and more so PTA, is often discussed because of the risks of "unnecessary" immunosuppression and surgical risks versus insulin, but solitary pancreas transplant extends many benefits to the recipient.[5,7] However, a review of the IPTR data found that the surgical risk was ameliorated at 4 years postoperatively, at which point mortality was equivalent to wait-listed patients.[28]

Multiple studies have also demonstrated the survival benefit of SPK versus kidney transplant alone in a recipient who has diabetes or an individual with diabetes on hemodialysis or who is wait-listed for SPK[7,13,28] One study argues that this benefit exists because the selected SPK recipients and donor organs were optimized for good outcomes. However, the investigators note that quality of life was not included in the outcome examination and that so including it may conclude superiority of the SPK.[15] A later study conducted by different investigators demonstrated that even if stratified by age, whereas patient survival was initially better in living donor kidney transplant alone in recipients who had diabetes, SPK patient survival was superior in cases of long-term (>10 y) graft survival.[29]

Although these pancreas transplant survival statistics are noteworthy, more important are the outcomes that were prevented or improved in their recipients. Pancreas transplantation restores euglycemia in a recipient with diabetes. This single achievement confers many secondary benefits. Diabetes is a risk factor for thrombosis because it is a hypercoagulable state, which may normalize a few months after successful pancreas transplantation.[19] Normalization of coagulation facilitates improvement of diabetic microvascular and macrovascular lesions.[13] These changes include a lower cumulative cardiovascular death rate[6,28–30] as well as stabilization or reversal of diabetic nephropathy with 5 years of normoglycemia [9,28,29] Addressing diabetic nephropathy may be among the most important aspects of a pancreas transplant because it potentially avoids the need for future kidney transplantation (or retransplantation as a result of reappearance of diabetic kidney lesions on the graft) if performed in the early stages of nephropathy,[5,9,13,30] as well as further reducing cardiovascular complications of renal disease.[28] Improvements in motor and autonomic neuropathy have also been described post–pancreas transplantation.[5,28,30]

Finally, and potentially most important to the recipient, pancreas recipients report improved quality of life in a newly euglycemic state.[7,15,29] Multiple studies report recipients of successful pancreas transplants report higher quality of life than their diabetic kidney transplant alone counterparts,[28] specifically in one study in the areas of physical and general health.[31] Thus, pancreas transplant has demonstrated patient survival benefit, physiologic improvement, and enhanced quality of life in recipients.

REFERENCES

1. Morath C, Schmied B, Mehrabi A, et al. Simultaneous pancreas-kidney transplantation in type 1 diabetes. Clinical Transplant 2009;23(Suppl 21):115–20.
2. Kelly WD, Lillehei RC, Merkel FK, et al. Allotransplantation of the pancreas and duodenum along with the kidney in diabetic nephropathy. Surgery 1966;61(6): 827–37.
3. Boggi U, Amorese G, Marchetti P. Surgical techniques for pancreas transplantation. Curr Opin Organ Transplant 2010;15:102–11.
4. Lillehei RC, Idezuki Y, Feemester JA, et al. Transplantation of stomach, intestine, and pancreas: experimental and clinical observations. Surgery 1967;62(4):721–41.
5. Kandaswamy R, Sutherland DER. Care of the pancreas transplant recipient. In: Irwin RS, Rippe JM, editors. Irwin and Rippe's Intensive Care Medicine. 6th edition. Philadelphia: Lippencott, Williams & Wilkins; 2007.
6. Gruessner AC, Sutherland DER, Gruessner RWG. Pancreas transplantation in the United States: a review. Curr Opin Organ Transplant 2010;15:93–101.
7. Lerner SM. Kidney and pancreas transplantation in type 1 diabetes mellitus. Mt Sinai J Med 2008;75(4):372–84.
8. Ohler L, Cupples S. Core curriculum for transplant nurses. St Louis (MO): Mosby Elsevier; 2008.
9. Fioretto P, Steffes MW, Sutherland DER, et al. Reversal of lesions of diabetic nephropathy after pancreas transplantation. N Engl J Med 1998;339:65–75.
10. Braunwald E, Fauci AS, Kasper DL, et al, editors. Harrison's Principles of Internal Medicine. 15th edition. McGraw Hill Publishing; 2001.
11. Centers for Disease Control and Prevention. National diabetes fact sheet: general information and national estimates on diabetes in the United States, 2005. Atlanta (GA): US Department of Health and Human Services, Centers for Disease Control and Prevention; 2005. Available at: http://www.cdc.gov/Diabetes/pubs/pdf/ndfs_2005. pdf. Accessed March 21, 2011.
12. Sheetz MJ, King GL. Molecular understanding of hyperglycemia's adverse effects of diabetic complications. JAMA 2002;288:2579–88.
13. Morath C, Zeler M. Transplantation in type 1 diabetes. Nephrol Dial Transplant 2009;24:2026–9.
14. Humar A, Ramcharan T, Kandaswamy R, et al. Technical failures after pancreas transplants: why grafts fail and the risk factors—a multivariate analysis. Transplantation 2004;78(8):1188–92.
15. Waki K, Terasaki PI. Kidney graft and patient survival with and without a simultaneous pancreas utilizing contralateral kidneys from the same donor. Diabetes Care 2006;29 (7):1670–2.
16. Conway P, Davis C, Hartel T, et al. Simultaneous kidney pancreas transplantation: patient issues and nursing interventions. ANNA J 1998;25(5):455–60, 478.
17. Stuart FP, Abecassis MM, Kaufman, DB. Organ transplantation. 2nd edition. Georgetown (TX): Landes Bioscience; 2003.

18. Goodman J, Becker YT. Pancreas surgical complications. Curr Opin Organ Transplant 2009;14(1):85–9.
19. Muthusamy AS, Giangrande PL, Friend PJ. Pancreas allograft thrombosis. Transplantation 2010;90(7):705–7.
20. Bass M, Galley-Reilley J, Twiss DE, et al. A diversified patient education program for transplant recipients. ANNA J 1999;26(3):287–92, 343.
21. Myers J, Pellino TA. Developing new ways to address learning needs of adult abdominal organ transplant recipients. Prog Transplant 2009;19(2):160–6.
22. Steinberg TG, Diercks MJ, Millspaugh J. An evaluation of the effectiveness of a videotape for discharge teaching of organ transplant recipients. J Transpl Coord 1996;6(2):59–63.
23. Schäfer-Keller P, Dickenmann M, Berry DL, et al. Computerized patient education in kidney transplantation: testing the content validity and usability of the Organ Transplant Information System (OTIS). Patient Educ Couns 2009;74:110–7.
24. Neyhart CD. Education of patient pre- and post-transplant: improving outcomes by overcoming the barriers. Nephrol Nurs J 2008;35(4):409–10.
25. Troppmann C. Complications after pancreas transplantation. Curr Opin Organ Transplant 2010;15(1):112–8.
26. Kauffman HM, Woodle ES, Cole EH, et al. Transplant recipient's knowledge of post-transplant malignancy risk: implications for educational programs. Transplantation 2008;85(7):928–33.
27. Drachenberg CB, Odorico J, Demetris AJ, et al. Banff schema for grading pancreas allograft rejection: working proposal by a multi-disciplinary international consensus panel. Am J Transplant 2008;8:1237–49.
28. Dean PG, Kudva YC, Stegall MD. Long-term benefits of pancreas transplantation. Curr Opin Organ Transplant2008;13(1):85–90.
29. Morath C, Zeier M, Döhler B, et al. Metabolic control improves long-term renal allograft and patient survival in type 1 diabetes. J Am Soc Nephrol 2008;19:1557–63.
30. Gremizzi C, Vergani A, Paloschi V, et al. Impact of pancreas transplantation on type 1 diabetes-related complications. Curr Opin Organ Transplant 2010;15(1):119–23.
31. Gross CR, Limwattananon C, Mathees B, et al. Impact of transplantation on quality of life in patients with diabetes and renal dysfunction. Transplantation 2000;70(12):1736–46.

Liver Transplantation: Issues and Nursing Care Requirements

Tracy A. Grogan, RN, MEd, BSN, CCRN, CCTN

KEYWORDS

• Liver • Transplantation • Nursing • Complications

More than 25,000 people die each year as a result of end-stage liver disease.[1] The term end-stage liver disease (ELSD) is a description as opposed to a specific diagnosis. A variety of specific illnesses can ultimately result in ESLD and multisystem organ dysfunction due to a failing liver. Many of these illnesses are also indications for liver transplant—the one treatment aimed at cure rather than symptom management. Liver transplant is not a panacea. The limited supply of organs will result in some patients not receiving a liver transplant. For those who do receive a liver transplant, the perioperative phase of liver transplantation will involve care and monitoring of all body systems.

INDICATIONS FOR LIVER TRANSPLANT

Hepatocytes are the functional units of the liver. Hepatocellular diseases injure or destroy hepatocytes, resulting in progressive liver failure. As the hepatocytes die, the liver tries to repair itself. However, the scarring and ultimate structural collapse of the liver leads to an ever decreasing number of functional hepatocytes and possible complications of bile drainage or blood flow due to the change in structure of the organ. Essentially any chronic ESLD that progresses to hepatic decompensation not controlled by medical management and acute liver failure may be an indication for liver transplant.[2] Clinical manifestations of hepatic decompensation include variceal bleeding, hepatic encephalopathy, ascites, spontaneous bacterial peritonitis, and hepatorenal syndrome.

Hepatocellular diseases that are indications for liver transplantation include alcohol-induced liver failure, chronic hepatitis, viral hepatitis, autoimmune hepatitis nonalcoholic steatorrhea hepatitis (NASH), and early-stage hepatocellular carcinoma. The Milan criteria are used to determine if the hepatocellular carcinoma is amenable to liver transplantation. Though there is some variation, patients with single lesions up

Transplant Intensive Care Unit, UPMC Presbyterian, University of Pittsburgh Medical Center, 200 Lothrop Street, Pittsburgh, PA 15213, USA
E-mail address: groganta@upmc.edu

Crit Care Nurs Clin N Am 23 (2011) 443–456
doi:10.1016/j.ccell.2011.08.002
0899-5885/11/$ – see front matter © 2011 Elsevier Inc. All rights reserved.

to 6.5 cm or not more than three lesions, each less than 3 cm, can be considered for liver transplantation.[3–5]

Cholestatic liver disease is another indication for liver transplant. Although produced by the liver, bile is also toxic to the liver. Normally, bile is contained and drained into the intestine by a network of ducts leading to the main bile ducts emptying into the intestine. Diseases such as primary biliary cirrhosis or primary sclerosing cholangitis alter the structural integrity of the biliary system, resulting in progressive liver failure.

Genetic and inborn errors of metabolism can be indications for liver transplantation. Disruptions in proteins such as cystic fibrosis, α_1-antitrypsin deficiency, amyloidosis, and maple syrup disease are conditions in which the liver itself may not fail but the liver dysfunction is the root cause of a compromised status of other vital organs.

Other diseases that can be indications for liver transplant include acute liver failure, veno-occlusive disease, fatty liver, cryptogenic cirrhosis, and childhood disorders such as biliary atresia.

THE GAP IN ORGAN SUPPLY AND DEMAND

Dr Starzl performed the first liver transplant in 1963. However, the issue of rejection was a major barrier in liver transplant being a viable and acceptable treatment for ESLD. The development of cyclosporine, a calcineurin inhibitor that blocks interleukin 2 synthesis by T lymphocytes, provided an effective immunosuppression resulting in allograft survival increasing to approximately 80%. As a result, the option of liver transplant became a viable and acceptable treatment for ESLD. Continued research into immunosuppressant agents resulted in more pharmacologic options for the management of rejection and achieving the goal of graft and host coexistence. This, coupled with improvements in surgical and anesthetic techniques such as low central venous pressure,[6] cell saver,[7] and antifibrinolytic agents,[8] have increased the 1-year survival rate for patients and liver allografts to approximately 87% and 82.7% respectively.[9]

There was rapid growth and refinement in liver transplant during the 1980s. In addition to immunosuppressive agents and management of rejection, surgical techniques were mastered that led to lower risks of the liver transplant operation and removed earlier contraindications for transplant such as portal vein thrombosis. More facilities began to offer liver transplant as an option so that the procedure became more available to patients across the United States as well as internationally. These improvements and increased accessibility were the beginning of the supply and demand imbalance for organs. Approximately 2 years ago there were 15,839 patients waiting for liver transplant (OPTN data as of May 13, 2009). The OPTN data as of April 30, 2010, almost 1 year later, posted 16,644 waiting for liver transplant. Across the United States 6320 liver transplants were performed in 2009 (OPTN data), yet the number of patients waiting increased by more than 800. Despite efforts to decrease the gap in organ supply and demand, the number of liver transplants performed throughout the United States has not significantly increased over the past 5 years.

Efforts to Expand the Organ Donor Pool

Several options to expand the number of organs for liver transplant are available. Extended criteria for use of cadaveric organs are possible as a result of medical and surgical advances.[10] This requires individualized scrutiny and assessment by the surgeon when matching an organ and a patient. Extended criteria include using organs that are hepatitis B core antibody positive (and treating the recipient to provide passive immunity), hepatitis C positive donors for hepatitis C positive recipients, donor organs with microvesicular steatosis, organs procured by donation after cardiac death,[11] and using organs from donors who were older than 65 years of age.

Domino transplant is another option used to expand the donor pool. The frequency in which domino transplant is an option may be low, but each incidence is yet another donor organ. Domino transplant can be used when a recipient is receiving a liver transplant because the native liver is the source of his or her illness, but the liver itself is not failing. Patients receiving transplant for errors in metabolism are potential candidates for their native liver to be "dominoed" to another recipient.

Donation after cardiac death is a strategy to expand the donor organ pool. The number of livers donated after cardiac death and used for transplant did rise, but these livers are associated with an increased risk of graft failure.[11] To maximize success with livers donated after cardiac death, the matching of the organ and the recipient must be carefully weighed by the surgeon.

Other options that help expand the donor pool include split liver transplant[12] and living donor liver transplants.[12–14] An example of a split liver is being able to split a donor liver large enough to accommodate the split to transplant the smaller left lobe into one recipient and the larger right lobe into another recipient. In a living donor liver transplant, a living person voluntarily undergoes a liver resection so that a portion of his or her liver that is large enough to initially sustain the recipient is removed and transplanted into the recipient. Both the living donor and the recipient need to have a liver portion that is large enough to support their bodies to allow for recovery and growth of the liver portions. Each will need to have a critical mass of healthy, functional hepatocytes (about 30% of normal liver). At the end of the healing and regeneration of the liver portions, both the donor and recipient will have at least 80% of "normal" liver size.

Isolated cases of using livers that have sustained severe injury as a result of blunt trauma for transplantation have been reported.[15–17] Using a severely injured liver for transplantation requires close scrutiny of the potential organ as well as the candidate for transplantation. Like several of the options for expanding the donor organ pool, this option can avoid wasting a viable organ, but is unlikely to significantly increase the number of donor organs.

Other efforts to expand the donor pool have not yet achieved practical clinical application. Cross-species transplant (xenograft), extracorporeal liver perfusion, artificial support, and bioartificial support have been investigated. A review of these options is provided elsewhere.[18]

Artificial (nonbiological) and bioartificial (hybrid) extracorporeal liver support has been a pursuit that, if successful, could help decompress the liver transplant waiting list. Artificial devices such as the molecular adsorbents recirculating system (MARS) and Prometheus systems, bioartifical devices using live hepatocytes, and hepatocyte transplant have been trialed in the clinical setting.[19] Bioartificial devices have used porcine hepatocytes and human hepatoblastoma cells artificially supported to serve as a bridge to transplant or in the case of acute liver failure a bridge to recovery. Successful cases have been achieved with each bioartificial device but none have demonstrated a significant decrease in patient mortality in clinical trials. The artificial systems have limited effect, as these systems are essentially albumin dialysis and lack the ability to synthesize proteins and perform other metabolic functions. A meta-analysis of artificial liver support suggests a 33% reduction in mortality when used for acute-on-chronic liver failure.[20] Because of the limitations of meta-analysis, this suggestion of decreased mortality would need to be validated.

Xenografts are yet another investigative alternative to the shortage of donor livers. In the past there have been attempts at ex vivo perfusion using pig livers in an effort to bridge patients to allotransplant and more recently using genetically engineered pigs to provide organs for xenotransplant. Although pig liver xenotransplant offers some advantages, there are still barriers to overcome before this becomes a reality.[18] Some of the advantages include an unlimited supply of organs, the ability to time the procedure to allow for a rested surgical team and medically optimize the patient, and higher assurance of a microbe-free organ. Issues still to be resolved include the coagulation dysfunction between pig and primate and preventing graft injury with prolonged immunosuppression.

TIMING OF LIVER TRANSPLANT

Determining when the risks of liver transplantation outweigh the risk of the waiting recipient's demise has been an area of intense focus. The US Department of Health and Human Services, surgeons, and the media have all voiced opinions on this issue. Ultimately the goal is to time the liver transplant when the patient's risk of dying within a relatively short time frame without the transplant exceeds the risk of death with only medical management.

Currently the Model for End-stage Liver Disease (MELD) scoring system is used to determine patient severity of illness and as an indicator of likelihood of death within the next 3 months.[3] Using a formula that uses the patient's current bilirubin, international normalized ratio, and creatinine, a patient receives a score. Scores range from 6 to 40, with 40 being the most severe illness. Consensus in the transplant community is that a score of 15 is the "breaking" point for the risk of transplant and the risk of continuing to wait. Most patients are considered for active listing to wait for transplant when the MELD score is 15 or greater. As a basis for allocation of deceased donor livers, the MELD scoring system has helped limit or eliminate some disparities in liver transplantation but not all.[21]

Use of objective criteria is a significant asset of the MELD scoring system. The limitation of the MELD score is that it is accurate only for the given time. The data have to be continually rechecked and the score recalculated to reflect a patient's current clinical status. The score can fluctuate in both directions over time dependent on the patient's liver function, overall health, or response to treatments. It is possible for a patient to have a relatively low MELD score but also have a poor clinical state, making the patient more acutely ill overall than reflected by the MELD score alone.[3]

OVERVIEW OF THE LIVER TRANSPLANT SURGICAL PROCEDURE

A detailed description of the standard technique for liver transplant surgery is found elsewhere.[2,22,23] After informed consent for the liver transplant surgery, anesthesia, and administration of blood products is completed the patient is taken to the operating area. Large-bore intravenous access and intravenous catheters required for invasive monitoring are inserted. The patient is intubated, anesthetized, and positioned on the operating room table. Proper positioning and attention to pressure relief are important factors to prevent complications such as circulatory compromise to an extremity, intraoperative or postoperative development of pressure-induced tissue injury, or peripheral nerve damage.

The surgery proceeds with the first incision usually resembling an inverted "Y". The liver is dissected and veins, arteries, and bile ducts are isolated. The vessels and bile ducts are clamped for removal of the native liver. The length of time and technical difficulty with the hepatectomy are dependent upon the existence of pathology. For example, portal hypertension preoperatively can result in a liver that is hard, making removal of the native liver more difficult. The extent of bleeding influences the duration and difficulty of the surgery. The presence of coagulopathy or the presence of dilated

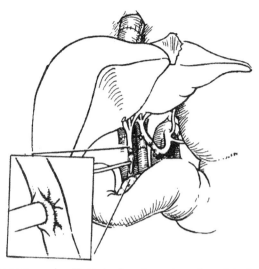

Fig. 1. Duct to duct anastomosis with t tube from transplantation of the liver. (*From* Klintmalm GB, Busuttil RW. The recipient hepatectomy and grafting. In: Busuttil RW, Klintmalm GB (eds). Transplantation of the liver. Philadelphia: WB Saunders;1996; with permission.)

and engorged vessels from portal hypertension may lead to significant blood loss and the need to reestablish hemostasis before continuing with surgery. Previous abdominal surgeries may have caused scar tissue, making dissection through the abdominal wall proceed slower and with more difficulty.

A second team of surgeons work on the donor organ as the recipient is undergoing the hepatectomy. This is often referred to as the "back table." It is essentially another operation being performed on the donor liver to prepare the organ for transplant. The donor organ blood vessels and bile ducts are inspected, repaired, and prepared for anastomosis with the recipient. The gallbladder of the donor liver is also removed.

On completion of the recipient hepatectomy and the donor organ preparation, the donor organ is placed into the recipient. Vessels are sewn together and there is close inspection for any leaks as clamps are removed. The donor organ is assessed for signs of good perfusion. When the vascular anastomoses are completed, the bile duct reconstruction is undertaken.

A duct-to-duct or choledochocholedochostomy procedure is used for bile duct reconstruction if the donor and recipient ducts are of adequate length (**Fig. 1**). Classically, choledochocholedochosotmy reconstruction occurs over a biliary stent or T-tube. Use of a T-tube offers some advantages, but is not without disadvantages.[24] Advantages of reconstruction over a T-tube include direct visualization of the bile, easy radiological access to the biliary tree, and more favorable prognostics for strictures. However, use of a T-tube is unfavorable regarding the occurrence of cholangitis and peritonitis.

A choledochojejunostomy (also called a Roux-en-Y) is performed when the portion of bile duct is too short for an end-to-end anastomosis. When the donor liver is harvested, surgical technique may result in shorter bile ducts. In the recipient the bile ducts may be affected by the patient's underlying disease (such as primary sclerosing cholangitis), and removal of diseased portions of the bile duct may result in a remaining length insufficient for end-to-end anastomosis. In this procedure, the bile ducts are connected directly into the intestine.

POSTOPERATIVE CARE AFTER LIVER TRANSPLANT

Since the early days of liver transplant, the core factors influencing recovery and essentials of immediate postoperative care have been consistent. Factors that influence recovery are the patient's pretransplant disease state and overall pretransplant clinical condition, quality of the donor organ, intraoperative events, and nursing care. Reviewing descriptions of nursing care in the immediate postoperative period show that, again, core components have remained over a 20-year span.[2,23,25]

The liver transplant procedure is lengthy and places a high degree of physiologic stress on the patient. Frequently patients are taken to the intensive care unit immediately after the surgery. As the patient is admitted, safe hand-off occurs as the surgical or anesthesia team or both describe the patient's medical/surgical history, events of the operation, and status of the body systems at the end of the procedure to the nurses and physicians in the ICU to whom the patient's care is transitioned.

An initial check of airway, breathing, and circulation occurs. Often nursing colleagues are working together so that assessments and tasks are performed simultaneously. If the patient is intubated, the endotube placement as well as ventilator settings and alarms are checked. Breath sounds are auscultated. Pulse oximetry is connected for ongoing monitoring. An arterial blood gas may be included in the initial assessment. Invasive monitoring lines are connected. Arterial and pulmonary artery (PA) catheter waveforms including central venous pressure (CVP) are assessed. Measurements of hemodynamic stability are taken: arterial blood pressure, cuff blood pressure, PA systolic and diastolic, and in many cases cardiac output and mixed venous saturation. Blood samples are sent to the laboratory for measurement of electrolytes, serum glucose, complete blood count (CBC), blood urea nitrogen (BUN), creatinine, bilirubin, and drug level for immunosuppressant agent; liver function tests (LFTs); and coagulation studies. A chest radiograph confirms position of the endotracheal tube and invasive monitoring lines and provides radiographic diagnostics for any pulmonary complications such as pulmonary edema or pleural effusion. All drains and tubes are checked initially for the quantity, color, and viscosity of drainage.

A second wave of assessment is performed immediately after safe hand off and the initial assessment for cardiopulmonary stability. Postoperative orders are reviewed. The initial postoperative orders usually include the laboratory values mentioned previously with repeat samples every 6 hours for the first 24 hours. Parameters for weaning the ventilator and for titration of any sedation, pain medications, or vasopressors are written. Other parameters may be included for laboratory results. Electrolyte replacement protocols, urine output, blood pressure (parameters for hypotensive and hypertensive patients), quantity of fluid from drains/tubes, hematocrit, and measurements of hemodynamic measurements from a PA catheter may have treatment orders for the nurse to initiate dependent upon the values.

A complete assessment ensues. Dependent upon the patient's temperature, this may be combined with bathing the patient in preparation for family visitation. Even in the absence of bathing, inspection of all skin surfaces should be integrated into the assessment process as patients are prone to pressure tissue injury after such a prolonged period of complete immobility. Any area that has redness or pallor or is slow to blanch should be considered an area of tissue pressure injury.

A head-to-toe assessment including all body systems in the context of the patient being immediate status post liver transplant is performed. It is important to remember that body systems function interdependently. This assessment is meant to determine the patient's baseline status for comparison for subsequent findings indicating

Table 1	
Early medical and surgical complications	
Surgical	**Medical**
Vascular (hepatic artery, portal vein, vena cava)	Preservation injury
Stenosis	Reperfusion injury
Occlusion	Pleural effusion
Leak	Infection
Biliary	Drug toxicity
Obstruction	Bleeding (coagulopathy)
Stenosis	Rejection
Leak	Impaired renal function
Liver infarction	
Surgical bleeding	
Diaphragm injury	

progress and function of the allograft or to detect complications including poor or declining allograft function. Early medical and surgical complications are listed in **Table 1**.

Neurologic

Initially, the neurologic exam is focused on monitoring for recovery from anesthesia. Mental status can be difficult to assess with anesthesia emergence. Pain with emergence from anesthesia can also complicate assessment findings. In the event that sedation or pain medication is needed, short-acting medications such as diprovan for sedation and fentanyl for pain are often used to facilitate frequent and accurate neurologic assessment without the effects of sedation or analgesic medications.

Seizure activity or failure to emerge from anesthesia are worrisome symptoms. Calcineurin inhibitors used for immunosuppression and metabolic abnormalities can produce a variety of neurologic symptoms including, but not limited to, confusion, dysphagia, psychosis, extrapyramidal symptoms, seizure, and coma. A patient can be having seizure activity or even status epilepticus without displaying muscle activity. For this reason, an electroencephalogram is often a diagnostic test ordered when a patient fails to emerge from anesthesia. Other diagnoses that need to be ruled out include encephalopathy, allograft failure or dysfunction, infection, cerebrovascular accident, and intracranial bleed.

Cardiovascular

In addition to monitoring hemodynamic parameters (blood pressure, cardiac output, PA, and CVP) patient laboratory values and vascular status need to be assessed. Again, metabolic imbalance can result in cardiac dysfunction and arrhythmias. Hypomagnesemia due to preoperative malnutrition, hypokalemia from flushing of the preserved liver intraoperatively, hyperglycemia from steroids or physiologic stress, hypertension, hypovolemia, and metabolic alkalosis are common problems in the immediate postoperative period. Often patients are in a hyperdynamic state pretransplant, and this state may remain in the early postoperative period. Left-side heart filling pressures help guide treatment for correction of intravascular fluid shifts. As the patient is rewarmed postoperatively, vasodilatation can create a picture of hypovolemia and transient hypotension.

Vascular complications may present as allograft dysfunction or be reflected in drainage from Jackson-Pratt (JP) drains or T-tube. Hepatic artery and portal vein thrombosis are potential but not common postoperative complications. Patency of these vessels is evaluated via Doppler ultrasound. Bleeding can be a result of an anastomosis leak, more superficial vessels that need to be cauterized or tied off, or inadequate correction of coagulation.

Pulmonary

The goal after liver transplant is early extubation (within the first 24 hours postoperatively). There are multiple potential complications that can impact the length of time the patient remains on ventilator support. As mentioned earlier, short-acting agents are used for sedation or analgesia if needed, as these medications will minimize the impact on length of intubation.

Oxygen availability and consumption may be continuously monitored using pulse oximetry and mixed venous saturation or intermittently via arterial blood gas sampling. Assessment of breath sounds and secretions is a priority. The liver transplant procedure requires prolonged anesthesia, supine positioning, and immobility. In addition, the patient may have had prolonged relative immobility due to failing health before transplant. As a result, atelectasis and accumulation and thicker secretions are common postoperative problems. Pleural effusions may result from postoperative fluid shifts and a poor nutritional state.

During the transplant procedure, the phrenic nerve may be injured, resulting in paresis or paralysis of the diaphragm (more often the right hemidiaphragm). Atelectasis, pleural effusion, metabolic alkalosis, and the abdominal incision may all contribute to a decrease in vital capacity.

In the early postoperative period bacterial infection is a common complication. Atelectasis, immobility, secretion management, and the presence of an artificial airway can all be predisposing factors to postoperative pneumonia. Nursing interventions such as oral hygiene, endotracheal tube care, early mobilization, patient positioning, and pulmonary toileting can help combat postoperative pneumonia. Bronchiole alveolar lavage can be performed at the bedside for diagnosis of infection or to clear deep thick secretions.

Gastrointestinal

Many complications following liver transplant are expected and readily managed. Ileus, mild gastric outlet obstruction, and ascites are complications following liver transplant surgery that may resolve without intervention. Stress ulceration is a potential complication after any major surgery or physiologic stressor. Prophylaxis is initiated in the immediate postoperative period. Nutritional compromise present preoperatively will persist in the initial postoperative period. This is reflected in amount of muscle mass and laboratory parameters such as serum albumin and urea nitrogen. It is important to initiate nutritional support as early as possible. For patients in whom early extubation is not achieved, enteral feedings should be initiated. Enteral feeding is preferred over central hyperalimination because enteral feeding can help stimulate bowel function and central hyperalimination can increase the incidence of postoperative infection.

Acute abdominal complications are relatively uncommon but vigilance with assessment for them is required for early intervention because these complications will have more immediate consequences to the patient and the new liver allograft. Often acute complications such as bowel perforation, biliary or vascular anastomosis leaks, and biliary or vascular stenosis require surgical intervention. Another acute but uncommon gastrointestinal complication is pancreatitis, requiring medical management. Intra-abdominal infection can occur, resulting in abscesses.

Liver allograft function is assessed in a variety of ways. Laboratory values are closely monitored. Elevated γ-glutamyltransferase and alkaline phosphatase levels can aid in identifying biliary complications. They are not in themselves diagnostic because other diagnoses such as sepsis, ischemic graft injury, reperfusion injury, and rejection can also elevate these laboratory values. Elevated aspartate aminotransferase (AST) and alanine aminotransferase (ALT) levels can be seen in poor or nonfunctioning allografts. A rising bilirubin level needs to be evaluated because this can indicate allograft dysfunction or a surgical complication or simply may be a rise reflective of corrected hemodilution or the patient having been transfused with red blood cells.

Characteristics of fluid from surgical drains can be an indicator of gastrointestinal complications or allograft dysfunction or both. If a T-tube is inserted, the bile (or lack of bile) can be observed. If the bile is anything other than a thick, stringy, dark green or golden brown further assessment is warranted. The absence of bile can indicate a kink in the drain occluding flow, occlusion of the bile duct, or a nonfunctioning allograft. The character of the fluid and the anatomic location of the drains can alert the nurse to complications (**Fig. 2**). Bloody JP drainage can indicate intraperitoneal bleeding. Cloudy drainage can be indicative of a bowel perforation. It is expected that JP drainage be thin and serosanguineous postoperatively. Stripping the JP drains will help prevent occlusion from fibrous tissue that may be present in the drain.

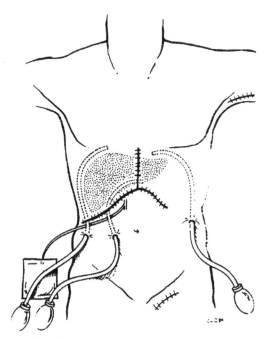

Fig. 2. Drain placement for liver transplantation. (*From* Klintmalm GB, Busuttil RW. The recipient hepatectomy and grafting. In: Busuttil RW, Klintmalm GB (eds). Transplantation of the liver. Philadelphia: WB Saunders;1996; with permission.)

Renal

There is a significant risk of renal insufficiency following liver transplantation. Even in the absence of renal pathology, many patients have renal insufficiency preoperatively. Perioperative events such as episodic or sustained periods of hypotension, hypovolemia, hemorrhage, antibiotic use, and immunosuppressive agents may contribute to renal insufficiency.

Renal function can impact management of volume shifts, third-space fluid, or pulmonary edema as well as electrolyte and metabolic balance. Close monitoring of urine output with accurate measurement via Foley catheter is required in the immediate postoperative period. The quality of urine is equally important. Insufficient creatinine clearance even in the presence of sufficient quantity will require intervention and support from renal medicine consultants. The calcineurin inhibitors used for immunosuppression can impair renal function.

Rejection

Rejection is a constant concern after transplant because rejection is the natural response of the immune system to a foreign body. Acute rejection is the most common type of rejection experienced by transplant recipients. If diagnosed and treated early, most cases of rejection are reversible. Acute rejection usually occurs within the first week to 3 months after transplant. On occasion, patients have presented with acute rejection years after transplant but this event is usually preceded by a manipulation in immunosuppression, for example, decreasing or discontinuing immunosuppression to manage an infection. This example demonstrates the importance of maintaining contact and a collaborative effort between a patient's primary care physician and the transplant center.

Chronic rejection occurs less frequently than acute rejection and over a much longer period of time. The ongoing process will ultimately lead to a state of end-stage liver failure and possibly the need for retransplant.

Signs and symptoms of rejection can vary.[2,22,23] Initially symptoms of rejection may be more general such as malaise, fatigue, loss of appetite, and low-grade fever. Differential diagnosis often includes infection. Liver-specific symptoms of rejection are similar to signs of liver failure and may include elevated liver enzymes, tenderness or pain over the liver, ascites, and jaundice. A liver biopsy is the only definitive objective test for rejection. However, a negative biopsy result does not automatically exclude the diagnosis of rejection. The liver is a large organ and the biopsy represents a very small sample of the liver. When all other diagnoses are ruled out, a patient may be treated for rejection based on clinical symptoms and laboratory data even in the absence of a liver biopsy demonstrating rejection.

Cellular rejection is more common than humoral rejection. Traditionally thought of as a potential early complication after transplant, humoral rejection can occur as a late complication even in the presence of rigorous compliance with the immunosuppressant regimen.[26]

If the liver biopsy demonstrates rejection, the rejection is graded using the Banff criteria.[22] The rejection is graded as mild, moderate, or severe based on the amount and extensiveness of cellular infiltration and inflammation. Hepatocytes may not be involved in mild rejection that is more evident in the epithelia of the central vein, sinusoids, and bile duct. This is due to the low expression of class I HLA on hepatocytes and the sinusoids, bile duct, and central vein epithelia having abundant class I and II major histocompatibility complex antigens.[23]

Recently there have been several theories related to the immunoprotective effect of the liver toward other donor-specific allografts. Starzl and colleagues found that some liver transplant recipients experienced graft survival without the use of immunosuppressants and ultimately proposed that donor-specific microchimerism could be induced through liver transplantation.[27] Fung and coworkers demonstrated kidneys with positive cross match results were protected from hyperacute rejection when the recipient simultaneously received kidney and liver transplants.[28] The hypothesis that the liver allograft is immunoprotective of other simultaneously transplanted allografts may not be unique to the liver. Other organ allografts such as the heart may also modulate the antidonor alloimmune response.[29]

Managing immunosuppression effectively is not the only intervention to try to avert rejection of the liver allograft. Postoperative serum glucose control has been shown to improve outcomes in critically ill patients. More recently, a retrospective review to evaluate if this held true in liver transplantation demonstrated an association between posttransplant hyperglycemia and increased risk of rejection.[30] Keeping the serum glucose below 200 mg/dL in the immediate postoperative period is another intervention to reduce the risk of rejection.

Infection

Infection is most likely the biggest risk factor after liver transplantation. Patients are twice as likely to have an episode of infection than an episode of rejection.[31] There are a sundry of contributing factors to infection following liver transplant. ESLD can lead to a debilitated clinical state, poor nutritional status, and derangement of the hepatic reticuloendothelial system and predispose the patient to infection after liver transplantation.[23] Other factors that contribute to increased risk of infection include receiving antibiotics within 2 weeks of transplant, previous multiresistant drug infections, pretransplant ascites, receiving hemodialysis after transplant, the need for reoperation after transplant, reactivation of recipient latent viruses, or transmission of organisms via the donor organ.[2,23,31]

In the immediate postoperative period, immunosuppression doses are the highest. This can give rise to opportunistic infections and infections from several sources (**Table 2**). It is important to control the factors that are within nurses' abilities to control, including monitoring hand washing of all health care providers and family/friends who enter the patient's room, monitoring housekeeping and cleaning of the room (many infections can survive on inanimate objects such as monitors, IV pumps, and bedrails), ensuring dressings are intact and cleaned appropriately, preventing body fluids from contaminating open wounds or incision sites, and bathing to help keep bacterial counts on the skin lower.

Table 2 Sources of infection		
Endogenous	Skin	Gram-negative bacteria
	Gastrointestinal tract	Gram-negative bacteria
	Latent viruses	Cytomegalovirus, Epstein–Barr virus, herpes simplex virus
Donor organ		Bacterial Viral
Environmental	Human	Bacterial, viral, fungal
	Water system	Bacterial
	Air system	Fungal
	Inanimate objects	Bacterial

Early infections after liver transplant (within the first 2–3 months) tend to be bacterial.[23,32] There are a variety of sites that make the transplant recipient vulnerable to bacterial infections including skin flora, abdominal drains, nasogastric tube, artificial airway, oral cavity, Foley catheter, venous and arterial catheters, and wounds, as these areas are typically colonized with bacteria. Oral hygiene, catheter care, skin care, tube care, and containment of body fluids can help prevent pneumonia and invasion of bacteria into the blood stream. Bacterial infection occurring after 3 months from transplant are more likely associated with a biliary source.[32]

Fungal and viral infections tend to be more opportunistic and occur later and are often the result of environmental exposure, reactivation of latent virus, and longer term immunosuppressive therapy. Many hospitals have construction projects within the hospital or in the immediate area that can increase the risk of early fungal infections in transplant recipients. When buildings are demolished, walls or ceilings invaded the risk of spores disseminating into the environment escalates. It is important that barriers be placed to prevent the infiltration of spores into the patient care environment, including spores being carried into the environment by health care workers, family, and construction workers.

The specific calcineurin inhibitor used to prevent rejection may not have a significant impact on whether or not infection occurs after liver transplant.[32] When investigating the infectious complications of liver transplant recipients receiving tacrolimus as the agent for immunosuppression, Singh and colleagues compared the results with previous studies investigating infectious complications following liver transplant in patients who received cyclosporine A as the immunosuppressant agent. Neither drug was associated with a higher incidence of infectious complications.

In part due to the immunosuppression that occurs at the time of transplant, not every patient with an infection will demonstrate all the "classic" signs of infection. Reid and colleagues found that most patients did not have fever and only half demonstrated leukocytosis when diagnosed with intra-abdominal infections in the early postoperative period.

To prevent infection, prophylaxis regimens are used. Antimicrobials such as ampicillin and cefotaxime or clindamycin and aztreonam for patients with penicillin allergies are usually administered for the first 24 hours postoperatively. Oral acyclovir can be ordered in low doses for prophylaxis of cytomegalovirus. Trimethoprim and sulfamethoxazole prophylax against pneumocystis. Dapsone or aerosolized pentamidine is substituted for patients allergic to sulfonamides.

SUMMARY

Liver transplantation has evolved into an accepted treatment for many suffering from end-stage liver failure. The complex nature of the liver results in every organ system being impacted by either the failing or the transplanted liver. Organ shortage remains problematic, and work to ensure maximizing the organ donor pool as well as the success of each organ transplant continues. The clinical care and condition of the patient before transplant can impact the outcome after transplant. Nurses can play an integral role in early identification of graft dysfunction, rejection, or infection. Because of the intimate and large amount of time that the nurse is at the patient's bedside, he or she is often in a position to monitor for potential risks to the patient and take corrective action.

REFERENCES

1. United Network for Organ Sharing. Available at: http://www.unos.org. Accessed April, 2010.
2. Rudow DL, Goldstein MJ. Critical care management of the liver transplant recipient. Crit Care Nurse Q 2008;31(3):232–43.

3. Selvaggi G. Patient selection in liver transplant: when is the right time to list? Mayo Clin Proc 2008;83(2):140–2.
4. Yao FY, Ferren L, Bass NM, et al. Liver transplant for hepatocellular carcinoma: expansion of the tumor size limits does not adversely impact survival. Hepatology 2001;33(6):1394–403.
5. Yao FY, Ferrel L, Bass NM, et al. Liver transplantation for hepatocellular carcinoma: comparison of the proposed UCSF criteria with the Milan criteria and the Pittsburgh modified TNM criteria. Liver Transpl 2002;8(9):765–74.
6. Massicotte L, Lenis S, Thibeault L, et al. Effect of low central venous pressure and phlebotomy on blood transfusion requirements during liver transplantation. Liver Transpl 2006;12:117.
7. Massicotte L, Thibeault L, Beaulieu D, et al. Evaluation of cell salvage autotransfusion utility during liver transplantation. HPB [Oxf] 2007;9:52.
8. Porte RJ, Molenaar IQ, Begliumini B, et al. Aprotinin and transfusion requirements in orthotopic liver transplantation: a multicenter randomized double-blind study. Lancet 2000;355:1303.
9. Scientific Registry of Transplant Recipients. Available at: http://ustransplant.org. Accessed April, 2010.
10. Renz JF, Kin C, Kinkhabwala M, et al. Utilization of extended donor criteria liver allografts maximizes donor use and patient access to liver transplantation. Ann Surg 2005;242(4):556–65.
11. Merion RM, Pelletier SJ, Goodrich N, et al. Donation after cardiac death as a strategy to increase decreased donor liver availability. Ann Surg 2006;244(4):555–62.
12. Humar A, Beissel J, Crotteau S, et al. Whole liver versus split liver versus living donor in the adult recipient – an analysis of outcome by graft type. Transplantation 2008; 82(10):1420–4.
13. Schemmer P, Mehrabi A, Friess H, et al. Living related liver transplantation: the ultimate technique to expand the donor pool? Transplantation 2005;80(15): 5138–41.
14. Fan ST. Live donor liver transplantation in adults. Transplantation 2006;82(6):723–32.
15. DiBenedetto F, Quintini C, DeRuvo N, et al. Successful liver transplantation using a severely injured graft. J Trauma Injury Infect Crit Care 2007;63(1):217–20.
16. Avolio AW, Agnes S, Chirico U, et al. Successful transplantation of an injured liver. Transplant Proc 2000;32:131–3.
17. Kraljevich M. Liver donation by a trauma patient: a case study in placement. J Transplant Coord 1999;9:153–5.
18. Elkser B, Gridelli B, Tector JA, et al. Pig liver xenotransplantation as a bridge to allotransplantation: which patients might benefit? Transplantation 2009;88(9): 1041–9.
19. Sgroi A, Serre-Beinier V, Morel P, et al. What clinical alternatives to whole liver transplantation? Current status of artificial devices and hepatocyte transplantation. Transplantation 2009;84(4):457–66.
20. Kjaergard LL, Liu J, Als-Nielsen B, et al. Artificial and bioartificial support systems for acute and acute-on-chronic liver failure. JAMA 2003;289(2):217–22.
21. Moylan CA, Brady CW, Johnson JL, et al. Disparities in liver transplantation before and after introduction of the MELD score. JAMA 2008;300(20):2371–8.
22. Abecasses M, Blei A, Koffron A, et al. Liver transplantation In: Stuart FP, Abecassis MM, Kaufman DB, editors. Organ transplantation. 2nd edition. Georgetown (TX): Landes Bioscience; 2003. p. 205–32.
23. Cosme M, Smith SL. Liver transplantation. Organ Transplant 2003. Medscape posted March 28, 2003.

24. Sotiropoulos GC, Sgourakis G, Radtke A, et al. Orthotopic liver transplantation: t-tube or not t-tube? Systematic review and meta-analysis of results. Transplantation 2009; 87(11):1672–80.

25. Whiteman K, Nachtmann L, Biondo M, et al. Liver transplantation. AJN 1990;June: 69–72.

26. Wilson CH, Agarwal K, Talbot D, et al. Late humoral rejection in a compliant ABO-compatible liver transplant recipient. Transplantation 2006;82(7):988–9.

27. Starzl TE, Demetris AJ, Trucco M, et al. Systemic chimerism in human female recipients of male livers. Lancet 1992;340:876–7.

28. Fung JJ, Makowka L, Griffin M, et al. Successful sequential liver-kidney transplantation in patients with preformed lymphocytotoxic antibodies. Clin Transpl 1987;1:187.

29. Rama A, Robles S, Russo M, et al. The combined organ effect: protection against rejection? Ann Surg 2008;248(5):871–9.

30. Wallia A, Parikh ND, Molitch ME, et al. Posttransplant hyperglycemia is associated with increased risk of liver allograft rejection. Transplantation 2010;89(2):222–6.

31. Reid GE, Grim SA, Sankary H, et al. Early intra-abdominal infections associated with orthotopic liver transplantation. Transplantation 2009;87(11);1706–11.

32. Singh N, Gayowski T, Wagener M, et al. Infectious complications in liver transplant recipients on tacrolimus. Transplantation 1994;58(7):774–8.

An Overview of Intestine and Multivisceral Transplantation

Mary Sheela Palocaren, RN, MSN, CCTN

KEYWORDS

- Intestine • Multivisceral • Transplantation • Nursing
- Complications

After the successful evolution of hepatic transplantation during the last decade, intestine and multivisceral transplantation remains the sole elusive achievement for the next era of transplant surgeons. Until recently, and for the last 30 years, the results of sporadic attempts at intestinal transplantation worldwide were discouraging because of unsatisfactory graft and patient survivals. The experimental and clinical demonstration of the superior therapeutic efficacy of tacrolimus, an immunosuppressive drug, ushered in the current era of intestine bowel and multivisceral transplantation with initial promising results.[1]

HISTORY

The first human bowel transplantation was performed in 1964 at the Boston Floating Hospital and 20 years later the first human multivisceral transplantation was done at the University of Pittsburgh. According to 1997 report of the International Registry, 33 intestinal transplant programs provided data on 273 transplants in 260 patients who were transplanted on or before February 28, 1997. The number of procedures per year has increased at a linear rate since 1990, with 58 transplants performed in 1996. Two thirds of the recipients were children or teenagers. Short gut syndrome or "gut failure" was the most common indication for transplantation. The types of transplants performed included the small bowel with or without the colon (41%), the small bowel and liver (48%), and multivisceral grafts (11%). The 1-year graft/patient survival for transplants performed after February 1995 was 55% to 69% for intestinal grafts, 63% to 66% for small bowel and liver grafts, and 63% for multivisceral grafts.[2]

By 2008, a total of 453 patients received 500 intestinal and multivisceral allografts. Of the 453 recipients, 198 (44%) received small bowel, 142 (31%) received combined liver–small bowel, and 113 (25%) received multivisceral grafts.[3]

Abdominal Transplantation, UPMC Presbyterian, University of Pittsburgh Medical Center, 200 Lothrop Street, Pittsburgh, PA 15213, USA
E-mail address: paloms@upmc.edu

Crit Care Nurs Clin N Am 23 (2011) 457–469
doi:10.1016/j.ccell.2011.08.003
0899-5885/11/$ – see front matter © 2011 Elsevier Inc. All rights reserved.

STATUS OF INTESTINE TRANSPLANTATION

Intestine transplantation has shown exceptional growth over the past 20 years with remarkable progress. University of Pittsburgh School of Medicine researchers assessed the evolution of intestine and multivisceral transplantation by reporting the first 500 such transplants conducted at the University of Pittsburgh Medical Center from 1990 to 2008, which represent more than 25% of the worldwide experience. Over nearly 2 decades divided into 3 eras, 453 patients received 215 small bowel, 151 liver–small bowel, and 134 multivisceral transplants. Some of these patients are the longest surviving small bowel and multivisceral transplant recipients in the world, surviving more than 19 years posttransplant with excellent quality of life.

During era I (1990–1994), transplant recipients were treated with the immunosuppressive drug tacrolimus and steroids. In 1994, this protocol was discontinued owing to high mortality and morbidity rates. The 5-year survival rate for these patients was 40%. Era II (1995–2001) introduced the use of donor bone marrow to encourage organ acceptance. The 5-year survival rate for these patients was 56%. During era III (2001–2008), patients underwent a preconditioning protocol with agents that deplete recipients' own immune calls. Their posttransplant drug regimen was minimal and was initiated with tacrolimus, followed by steroids when necessary. Tacrolimus doses were subsequently spaced to a single dose twice to 3 times per week with a careful weaning process that started 3 to 6 months posttransplantation. Through the use of new immunosuppressive and management strategies, the 5-year survival rate for these patients increased to 68%, which is similar to any other abdominal and thoracic organ transplant procedure.[3]

Living donor bowel transplantation has recently emerged as a valuable alternative to cadaver bowel transplant. Most of the intestinal transplants have been performed using intestinal graft obtained from cadaver donors. The use of living donor bowel grafts can add some important advantages with acceptable risks for the donors. To date, only 32 small bowel transplants (3.3% of the total) have been performed from living donor versus 957 from deceased donors. Living donor intestinal transplantation offers substantial potential advantages that make it theoretically quite attractive. This strategy makes the transplant an elective procedure with minimization of waiting time, reduces cold ischemia time, and allows human leukocyte antigen matching.[4]

INDICATIONS

For nearly 3 decades, the small bowel was considered a forbidden organ for transplantation because of the associated massive lymphoid tissue, high antigenicity, and microbial colonization. With the clinical introduction of effective immunosuppressive agents, the risk of allograft rejection and the lethal host infection were ameliorated and the procedure has become a clinical reality.[5] Patients with chronic intestinal failure are candidates for small bowel transplant either alone, combined with the liver, or as part of a multivisceral graft that includes stomach, duodenum, pancreas, and small bowel with or without the liver.

Isolated Small Bowel Transplantation

Short bowel syndrome or "gut failure" is the most common indication for isolated small bowel transplantation. The primary causes are as follows.

Crohn's disease

Chronic inflammation of the small bowel that can involve multiple segments of the gastrointestinal (GI) tract. The disease may be severe and require multiple extensive bowel resections, resulting in dependence on total parenteral nutrition (TPN).

Intestinal vascular insufficiency

Intestinal vascular insufficiency results from motor vehicle accidents, gunshot wounds, or other types of trauma. It is also precipitated by hypercoagulable states, such as factor V mutation, protein C, S or antithrombin III deficiencies, or the presence of lupus anticoagulant or anticardiolipin antibodies. Budd–Chiari syndrome is another vascular abnormality that has wide range of presentations, from a venous occlusive disorder with small vessel occlusion to thrombosis of the major hepatic veins and/or the inferior vena cava.[6]

Hereditary/congenital disorders

Familial adenomatous polyposis is an autosomal-dominant disorder characterized by the development of the polyps in the large small bowel. Gardner's syndrome is a form of familial adenomatous polyposis that includes intestinal polyposis as well as soft tissue tumors and osteomas. A further complication of polyposis is the development of desmoid tumors or diffuse mesenteric fibromatosis.[7]

Radiation damage

Radiation therapy may cause radiation enteritis. Patients present with bloody diarrhea and rectal bleeding, and eventually develop malabsorption syndrome. Inflammation, ulceration, and fistula formation are seen on endoscopy and the intestinal biopsy reveals villous atrophy with focal to progressive fibrosis.[8]

Combined Liver and Small Bowel Transplantation

Patients with short bowel syndrome and TPN-associated hepatic failure are candidates for combined liver and small bowel transplantation. The replacement of both organs is also the only technically feasible and safe procedure that can be offered to the liver failure patients with associated portomesenteric venous thrombosis.

Multivisceral Transplantation

Full or modified multivisceral transplantation is indicated for patients with massive GI polyposis, traumatic loss of the abdominal viscera, extensive abdominal desmoid tumors, locally aggressive nonmetastasizing neoplasms, and complete thrombosis of the splanchnic arterial or portal venous system with vascular or hepatic decompensation.[5]

CONTRAINDICATIONS

Contraindications are either relative or complete and include, but are not limited to cardiopulmonary insufficiency, incurable malignancy, persistent life-threatening intra-abdominal or systemic infections, and severe immune deficiency syndromes. A remote history of GI malignancy, the presence of respectable desmoid or stromal tumors, and active abdominal infections at the time of referral should not be considered as absolute contraindications for transplantation.[5]

RECIPIENT SELECTION

Patients with no jejunoileum who have certain lifelong parenteral dependence, should be immediately referred to a transplant center owing to the high likelihood of the development of liver disease. Patient criteria include the following: (1) Adequate cardiovascular function (ejection fraction greater than or equal to 40%); (2) absence of acute or chronic active infections that are not effectively treated, (3) no uncontrolled and/or untreated psychiatric disorders that interfere with compliance to a strict treatment regimen, (4) no active alcohol or chemical dependency that interferes with compliance to a strict treatment regimen. Persons with a history of drug or alcohol abuse must be abstinent for at least 3 months before being considered a transplant candidate eligible for coverage. (5) Absence of inadequately controlled HIV or AIDS defined as a CD4 count greater than 200 cells/mm^3 for longer than 6 months, HIV-1 RNA (viral load) undetectable, on stable antiviral therapy for longer than 3 months, no other complications from AIDS, such as opportunistic infections (eg, aspergillus, tuberculosis, *Pneumocystis carinii* pneumonia, toxoplasmosis encephalitis, crypto-coccal meningitis, disseminated coccidioidomycosis, other resistant fungal infec-tions), or neoplasms (Kaposi sarcoma, non-Hodgkin's lymphoma). Preoperative evaluation requires a complete multidisciplinary assessment to clearly define the cause of isolated intestinal or intestinal/hepatic failure.

DONOR SELECTION

Hemodynamically stable, heart-beating diseased donors who have no intestinal pathology represent the majority of the donors. Cytomegalovirus (CMV)-positive donors are accepted for CMV-positive recipients.[9]

POSTOPERATIVE COMPLICATIONS
Hemorrhage

Hemorrhage is usually related to a technical problem from an anastomotic leak, peritoneal bleeding, or vascularized adhesions from previous surgeries. Preexisting coagulopathy and portal hypertension may predispose patients with hepatic dysfunc-tion to bleed. Symptoms include Pallor, tachycardia, hypotension, increased drainage through Jackson–Pratt drains, reduction in serial hemoglobin levels, abnormal serum pH, and lactate levels may indicate intestinal ischemia or tissue injury. Treatment is with operative reexploration and repair; administration of blood products contributes to the resolution of the bleeding.[10]

Biliary

Biliary complication usually occur in the early postoperative period and may be seen in combined small bowel/liver grafts. Symptoms include leakage through the abdom-inal wound and/or bilious fluid in the surgical drains.[10] Treatment consists of reexploration and repair of the dehiscence, or revision of the anastomosis.

Vascular

These are rare, but significantly compromise the graft and result in necrosis of the organs perfused by that arterial supply. Symptoms include significant elevation of hepatic enzymes, the stoma may become pale or dusky, the function of the graft deteriorates, sepsis, and fulminant liver failure. Standard therapy with anticoagulants decreases the risk of thrombus; surgical intervention, including enterectomy (removal of the small bowel graft, is another option.

GI

Leaks from the proximal and distal anastomosis may occur within the initial postop-erative period owing to technical problems or poor wound healing secondary to immunosuppression and malnutrition. Confirmation of the leakage is obtained by contrast imaging. Symptoms include abdominal distention, fever, and peritonitis. Prevention and treatment consist of decompression of the small bowel through the jejunostomy, ileostomy, and nasogastric tube to minimize the risk of leaks. Surgical exploration to revise the affected segment of small bowel and remove the infected peritoneal fluid is required, in addition to a full course of intravenous (IV) antibiotics and/or antifungal therapies.

GI Bleeding

Early bleeding occurs owing to technical problems and may require surgical intervention. Late bleeding may be a sign of rejection or infection. Endoscopy and biopsy are required to definitively diagnosis an infectious etiology versus rejection. Symptoms include sanguineous ileostomy drainage or rectal bleeding, tachycardia, hypotension, abdominal pain, and decreasing hemoglobin levels.[10] Surgical intervention is necessary for technical problems; however, if the etiology is rejection, then the treatment is increased immunosuppression, or if it is infection, antimicrobials and reduced immunosuppression.

Hypermotility

This is common in the early posttransplant period. Peristalsis begins when the small bowel is reperfused, but can be erratic. Fluid and electrolyte balance must be accurately maintained by monitoring intake and output, daily weight, and serum electrolytes.

POSTOPERATIVE NURSING CARE

Management of the intestine transplant recipient is a complex and formidable task, particularly during the first 6 months posttransplantation. These patients are vulnerable to a wide range of complications related to rejection, infection, and technical problems. The greatest challenge is achieving a balance between adequate amounts of immunosuppression to prevent rejection while avoiding a heavy-handed approach that may result in infectious complications. It is imperative that medical management includes surveillance studies with a preventative approach to early detection and treatment. Foremost, a multidisciplinary approach is required for an optimal outcome through the teamwork of transplant surgeons, GI specialists, infectious disease specialists, nursing staff, psychologists, social workers, and occupational and physical therapists, as well as an array of other consultants. Intestine transplant recipients are require meticulous medical management with consistent long-term follow-up care.

Fluid and Electrolyte Balance

The body obtains its daily requirements of fluid and electrolytes through absorption from the GI tract. Fluids and electrolytes are vital for the body's function, both metabolically and cellularly. After surgery, fluid and electrolyte requirements are different from the normal state for several reasons: Additional fluid loss through drains, stomas, and nasogastric tubes increase the amount of the electrolytes that the body will lose, and the release of intracellular potassium from cells damaged during surgery may cause a transient rise in serum levels. Consequently, there is a dynamic balance that requires careful monitoring to ensure that daily maintenance needs are met and the serum concentration is maintained.[11]

Nursing responsibilities

- Maintain strict record of intake and output.
- Observe for symptoms of electrolyte imbalance, fluid overload or dehydration.
- Obtain electrolytes and renal function tests as ordered.
- Notify physicians regarding abnormal laboratory results.
- Administer IV fluids to correct imbalances as ordered.
- Obtain repeat laboratory values to evaluate decree of imbalance.
- Weigh patient daily at the same time and on the same calibrated scale.
- Monitor vital signs and report abnormalities.
- Observe for neurologic changes.

Pain Management

Effective postoperative pain control is an essential component of the care of the surgical patient. Inadequate pain control, apart from being unfeeling, may result in increased morbidity or mortality. Evidence suggests that surgery suppresses the immune system and that this suppression is proportionate to the invasiveness of the surgery.[12] Pain can have devastating effects on patients and families. In the words of ethicist Edwin Lisson, "Disease can destroy the body, but pain can destroy the soul."[13] The ethical responsibility to control pain and relieve suffering is at the core of the health care professional's commitment to the patient.[14] Pain is a significant clinical problem where nursing care absolutely matters.[15]

Nursing responsibilities

- IV patient-controlled anesthesia.
- Oral narcotics are prescribed when patients are tolerating the enteral feeds.
- Assess patient for excessive sedation, respiratory depression, bradycardia, and hypotension.
- Assess the graft for dysmotility; constipation is a side effect of narcotics and motility of the transplanted intestine may be further compromised with prolonged narcotic use.
- Provide patients with information on the importance of pain management to maintain mobility and safety, and address patient's fears of addiction.[16]

Enteral Feeding

Postoperative hyperalimentation, such as TPN and/or enteral nutrition is often required in the early postoperative period until mucosal function impaired by ischemia and reperfusion recovers.[17] A number of physiologic adjustments are required of the transplanted bowel before satisfactory intestinal function occurs. Enteral feedings are started when the bowel sounds are present. The enteral feed is initially given slowly and continuously over a 24-hour period to enhance absorption. Bolus feeds are introduced later.[18]

Nursing responsibilities

- Evaluate the feeding system, including the container of the formula and the delivery set to prevent contamination.
- Wash hands and wear nonsterile disposable gloves before assembling and handling any part of the feeding system.
- With open systems, avoid adding new formula to that remaining in the container from previous administration.[19]

- Use sterile water for dilution and irrigation because the patient is immunocompromised.
- Maintain irrigation sets with medical asepsis and replace them every 24 hours.
- Prevent aspiration by keeping the head of the bed at 30° to 45° at all times.[20]
- Stop the feeding and flush the tube before administration of medication.
- Medication must be administered separately. Irrigate the feeding tube with water before and after each medication.[21]
- Use elixir/suspension modes of medication when possible.[22]
- Restart the feeding in a timely manner to avoid compromising nutritional status.

Stoma Care

An ileostomy is created to provide access to the transplanted intestine for routine surveillance, including biopsy, for rejection. The bulk of stool output drains from the ileostomy and the drainage is emptied and recorded. Stool is assessed for amount, color, and consistency; consistency is watery in the early period because the large intestine is bypassed. As motility stabilizes, the stool output will be 1 to 2 L/d in adults. Peristomal skin protection is the cornerstone of ostomy management; treatment of the skin relies on methods to create dry surfaces, fill irregular contours, and treat infections; an adhesive seal is maintained.[23]

Nursing responsibilities

- Assess the stoma postoperatively for any clinical manifestations of necrosis.
- Assess skin for erythema and signs of breakdown during pouch change.[24]
- Apply skin barrier to protect skin from intestinal contents.
- Empty pouch when it is one third full to prevent the seal from leaking.
- Gentle removal of adhesives is recommended to avoid skin stripping. The pouching system is removed by supporting the skin and using a soft tissue with water.
- Maintaining dry skin reduces the risk of developing candidiasis and is critical to obtaining a good adhesive seal.
- Teach patient proper skin and appliance care to ensure proper technique for long-term care.
- Plan for outpatient or home visit for continued teaching.

Monitoring Graft Function

The creation of an ileostomy at the time of transplantation is critical for its use in monitoring the function of the graft, performing endoscopy, and obtaining biopsy specimens. Graft function must be monitored daily in the early postoperative period.[25] The character of the graft stoma is assessed frequently for texture, color, and friability. Stomal output is assessed for volume, consistency, blood, and pH. Endoscopic evaluation of the graft is performed via the graft ileostomy and via upper GI endoscopy. Mucosal biopsies are also taken according to center-specific protocols. Intestinal absorption of D-xylose and tacrolimus assessed as evidence of graft function.

Nursing responsibilities

- Observe for abdominal distention and signs of discomfort or pain.
- Auscultate for hypoactive bowel sounds.
- Palpate to assess any firmness or abdominal rigidity.
- Assess stoma output for any changes:

- Volume: Acute increase in stoma output.
- Color: From yellowish-brown to melena and/or rank blood.
- Consistency: Increased watery fluid with little consistency.

ACUTE REJECTION EPISODES

Rejection is a common complication after intestine transplantation because of the large amount of lymphoid tissue associated with the graft. To monitor for possible development of acute rejection, surveillance endoscopies are performed once or twice per week during the early postoperative period.

Symptoms

Symptoms of acute rejection include fever, abdominal distention, cramping, vomiting, abdominal pain, any change in the appearance of the stoma, and a significant increase or decrease in stool output.

Endoscopic Findings

Mild to moderate rejection is characterized by localized inflammatory infiltrate, intact mucosa, erythema/or duskiness, loss of normal velvety appearance, and absent or decreased peristalsis. Severe rejection is characterized by crypt damage and mucosal ulceration and denuded mucosa with bleeding.

Histologic Findings

Histologic findings include acute rejection includes increased apoptotic bodies, the presence of activated lymphocytes, loss of goblet cells, blunted villae, and ulceration.[26] With severe rejection, the crypts between the villae are destroyed and the epithelium is sloughed.

Treatment

Treatment of mild to moderate rejection includes administering IV methylprednisolone as a bolus dose with decreasing cycled dosing over a short period of time, optimizing tacrolimus levels, and adding adjunctive agents to the baseline immunosuppressive regimen. Repeat biopsies assess the effect of treatment and determine further management. For severe rejection, alternate treatment (1–4 doses) with rabbit antithymocyte globulin (Thymoglobulin) is initiated. The duration of therapy determined by subsequent histology. Consider graft enterectomy if the rejection episode is refractory to all available treatments and the patient has increased complications related to infections from high levels of immunosuppression.

INFECTIONS

Patients who undergo intestinal transplantation are more susceptible to infectious complications than other transplant recipients. The heavy immunosuppression required to prevent intestinal allograft rejection places the patients at a higher risk for the development of infections. The major posttransplant infections include CMV, Epstein-Barr virus (EBV), adenovirus, and bacterial and fungal infections. Because these infections can be confused clinically with other causes of intestinal allograft dysfunctions, including acute rejection episodes, accurate diagnosis is critical for patient management.

CMV

CMV infection occurs in approximately one third of the patients receiving intestine allografts.[27] The primary disease occurs in patients who were seronegative before transplantation and became infected with a latent virus from a CMV-seropositive donor. CMV infection can be characterized by a self-limiting syndrome of episodic fever spikes for a period of 3 to 4 weeks, arthralgias, fatigue, anorexia, abdominal pain, diarrhea, and focal ulcerations of the intestine with bleeding.[28] Techniques for rapid diagnosis of CMV infection include shell vial culture, pp65 antigenemia assay, polymerase chain reaction, and the hybrid-capture RNA–DNA hybridization assay for qualitative detection of CMV-polymerase chain reaction. Recently, attention has been focused on the role of the quantitative CMV viral load as an accurate diagnostic test for CMV. Although in general CMV viral load correlates with viral disease, CMV disease can occur in the setting of a very low viral load. In addition, viral load is an optimal parameter to use for monitoring response to antiviral therapy.[29]

Prevention of CMV infection is the standard of care in transplant recipients. Ganciclovir is most commonly used for the prevention of CMV infection in intestine transplant recipients. Ganciclovir is administered either IV or orally, and either as general prophylaxis or as part of a preemptive strategy.[29]

EBV

EBV may infect the B cells, either from primary EBV virus transmitted from the donor or as a result of a reactivation of the virus posttransplantation. Organ transplant recipients are at increased risk for diseases caused by the EBV. The majority of these diseases, known collectively as B-cell lymphoproliferative disorders or posttransplant lymphoproliferative disease (PTLD), when present in transplant recipients, are EBV-associated and frequently occur within the first year following transplantation. Intestine transplant recipients are at a relatively high risk of developing PTLD compared with other organ transplant populations with approximately 20% of patients with intestine allografts diagnosed with PTLD.[25]

Because higher levels of immunosuppression are prescribed for intestinal transplant patients, there is a greater incidence of PTLD and it occurs earlier than in other types of transplantation. Because primary EBV infection is a risk factor for the development of PTLD, it is essential to identify patients at risk by performing EBV serology before transplantation.[30] The patients at greatest risk for developing PTLD are EBV-seronegative recipients who received EBV-seropositive organs. After transplantation, those patients should be carefully monitored for the acquisition of EBV infection.[31]

PTLD is a neoplastic disease and a progressive increase in therapy is implemented after diagnosis. It begins with a reduction of immunosuppression for low-grade PTLD, continues with anti-CD20–directed rituximab therapy against higher grade of PTLD, and ends in treatment using recognized non-Hodgkin's lymphoma protocols in cases of highly aggressive PTLD.[32] PTLD is a major cause among death intestine transplant recipients.[33] Preventive strategies, early detection, and aggressive treatment of PTLD are essential to decrease the morbidity and mortality of this complication of immunosuppression.[29]

Graft Versus Host Disease

Graft versus host disease (GVHD) is recognized as a potential complication after intestine transplantation because the large inoculums of lymphoid cells in the small bowel graft are predicted to increase the likelihood of this disease.[34] GVHD occurs in approximately 5% of patients undergoing intestine transplantation, a rate that is 5 to 10 times greater than in other solid organ transplant recipients.[25]

The diagnosis of GVHD is based on both clinical presentation and histopathologic confirmation. Suggestive clinical signs and symptoms include mild pruritis and an initial skin eruption, usually a macular erythematous rash present on the upper trunk, neck, and feet. Macular and papular areas may coalesce and form confluent areas of involvement; blisters may occur, particularly on the palms, soles, and the abdominal skin. Other clinical manifestations may include mouth or tongue lesions, perianal rash or eczema, diarrhea, native GI tract ulceration, native liver dysfunction, and bone marrow suppression, including pancytopenia.[32]

Bacterial Infections

Most bacterial infections are caused by organisms that are previously colonized in the patient and originate at sites of mucosal damage. Bacterial infections generally begin when bacteria bypass local anatomic and mechanical defense mechanisms. In addition to the observable examples of a break in the skin or the insertion of invasive catheters, another important mechanism of bacterial infection is the loss of the gut mucosal barrier. The gut serves as a primary reservoir for life-threatening bacteria in immunosuppressed individuals. The common organisms are *Enterobacter*, *Klebsiella*, *Pseudomonas*, polymicrobial infections, and antibiotic-resistant organism such as vancomycin-resistant enterococcus.

Signs and symptoms of bacterial infections are fever above 101°F (38.5°C); flu-like symptoms (malaise, lethargy, decreased appetite); catheter or tube insertion sites that are erythematous, swollen, or tender (the wound site may exhibit erythema, purulent drainage, tenderness, or swelling); wound dehiscence; changes in respiratory status including tachypnea, decreased breath sounds, or cough; and changes in drainage, such as purulence, cloudy urine, or a change in stool consistency and odor. The infection is diagnosed through central and peripheral cultures, and wound, drain, urine, and stool testing. A chest x-ray (if patient has respiratory symptoms), and abdominal computed tomography can be used to identify the source of infection. The treatment protocol is initially treatment with broad spectrum antibiotics; then, antimicrobials are prescribed based on the sensitivity of the identified organisms.

Bacterial Pneumonia

Administer IV antibiotics as ordered, monitor oxygen flow and oxygen saturation, encourage coughing, deep breathing, and incentive-spirometry, and encourage the patient to ambulate.

Central Line Infection

The line may be removed, the patient treated with IV antibiotics, and blood cultures monitored until negative.

Fungal Infections

Despite ongoing refinements in immunosuppressive agents, graft preservation, and operative techniques, fungal infections remain a significant cause of morbidity and mortality among organ transplant recipients. The advent of effective antibacterial and antiviral prophylactic and therapeutic strategies has led to the emergence of opportunistic mycoses as a principal cause of infection-related mortality among organ transplant recipients.

Candida and *Aspergillus* species have accounted for most invasive fungal infections in organ transplant recipients. The frequency of fungal infections and the time of onset of infection differ for various types of solid organ transplants. *Candida* infections occur most frequently in liver, pancreas, and intestine transplant recipients, whereas the impact of invasive aspergillosis is greater among lung and liver transplant recipients.[35]

Invasive fungal infections have been reported in 40% to 59% of the intestine transplant recipients; most are caused by invasive *Candida* species.[35] Disruption in the integrity of the GI tract, the requirement of relatively higher immunosuppression, and an unusually high incidence of CMV infection in these patients may account for a higher incidence of *Candida* infections in intestine transplant recipients.[33]

Candida infections are generally derived from endogenous flora. Candida species observed in transplant recipients include *C albicans*, *C glabrata*, *C tropicalis*, *C parapsilosis*, *C krusei*, *C lustitaniae*, *C rugusa*, *C kefyr*, and *C guilliermendii*. *C albicans* ranks as the most common species, with *C glabrata* and *C tropicalis* emerging as other causative pathogens. Candida syndromes include mucocutaneous infection, pneumonia, empyema, wound infection, esophagitis, abdominal infection (tissue infection of the liver, spleen, or pancreas; peritonitis; abdominal abscesses either as a sole pathogen or in a polymicrobial infection; enteritis), candiduria, pyelonephritis, fungal ball formation within the genitourinary system or preexisting pulmonary cavity, catheter- or foreign body-associated candidiasis, candidemia (transient or with associated sepsis), endocarditis, brain abscess, meningitis, endophthalmitis, chorioretinitis, sinusitis, and musculoskeletal disease (osteomyelitis, chondritis).

Aspergillus

Species of medical importance include *Aspergillus fumigatus*, *A flavus*, *A niger*, *A terreus*, *A nidulans*, *A glaucus*, *A ustus*, *A versicolor*, *A oryzae*, *A sydowi*, and *A chevalieri*. *Aspergillus* infections may include 1 or more *Aspergillus* species from an individual patient.[36] CMV prevention strategies and induction protocols using anti-lymphocyte therapy may affect the incidence of *Aspergillus* infection. *Aspergillus* spores are ubiquitous and are frequently isolated from hospital ventilation systems, especially during periods of construction or renovation; community environmental exposures may also occur. Inhalation of fungal spores is the primary mode of acquiring *Aspergillus*; therefore, the lung and upper respiratory tract are the most common sites of occurrence.

Aspergillus syndromes include invasive pulmonary disease, tracheobronchitis, empyema, necrotizing pneumonia, disseminated disease with central nervous system involvement (brain abscess, infarction, endophthalmitis), and rhinosinusitis. Other manifestations of disease include isolated visceral involvement (liver, kidney, spleen, GI tract, myocardium, thyroid, testicle, prostate, and pericardium); angiotropic invasion with thrombosis and infarction; GI involvement; fungal ball formation in preexisting cavities, sinuses, genitourinary conduits, and the bladder; osteomyelitis; and primary or disseminated cutaneous disease.

Antifungal Prophylaxis

Prophylactic or preemptive antifungal strategies are controversial, and approaches vary among different transplant programs. Antifungal prophylaxis has been based on individual risk factors, the incidence of fungal infections at a particular center, clinical experience, and specific posttransplant complications.[37]

Three types of antifungal strategies have been described: Therapeutic, prophylactic, and preemptive approaches. Therapeutic use refers to treatment of an established infection; prophylactic use involves administration of an agent to all recipients to prevent infection; and preemptive use involves administration of an agent to a subgroup of recipients determined to be high risk as defined by clinical, laboratory, or epidemiologic characteristics.

Antifungal agents should possess characteristics, including rapid fungicidal activity, favorable pharmacokinetics and bioavailability, low to absent toxicity to the allograft and other organ function, and minimal or predictable interactions with concurrent immunosuppressives, particularly calcineurin inhibitors.

SUMMARY

Intestine transplantation remains a formidable clinical and immunologic challenge. With newer immunosuppressive agents and accumulated experience, the survival outcomes for these patients are improving. The relationship of recipient preexisting conditions with the risk of postoperative events clearly emphasize the necessity of early referral of patients with intestinal failure to expert transplant program before the onset of life-threatening complications.[30] With increased awareness and knowledge regarding referral criteria, transplant criteria, optimal time for transplantation, and medication regiments, improved patient outcomes after intestine and multivisceral transplant will be achieved.

REFERENCES

1. Abu-Elmagd K, Todo S, Tzakis A, et al. Three years clinical experience with intestinal transplantation. J Am Coll Surg 1994;179(4):385–400.
2. Grant D. Intestinal transplantation: 1997 Report of the International Registry. Transplantation 1997; 67 (7):1061–4.
3. Abu-Elmagd K, Costa G, Bond GJ, et al. Five hundred intestinal and multivisceral transplantations at a single center. Annals of Surgery 2009;250(4):567–81.
4. Benedetti E, Holterman M, Asolati M, et al. Living related segmental bowel transplantation. Ann Surg 2006;244(5):694–9.
5. Abu-Elmagd K. Intestinal transplantation: indication and patient selection. In: Langnas AN, Goulet O, Quigley EMM, et al, editors. Intestinal failure: diagnosis, management and transplantation. New York: Blackwell; 2008. p.245–53.
6. Glenn M, Todo S, Tzakis A, et al. Liver transplantation for the Budd-Chiari syndrome. Ann Surg 1990;211:43–9.
7. Winter HS. Intestinal polyps. In: Walker WA, Durie PR, Hamilton JR, et al, editors. Pediatric gastrointestinal disease: pathophysiology, diagnosis, management. 2nd edition. St Louis: Mosby; 1996. p. 891–906.
8. Kelijo DJ, Squires RH. Anatomy and anomalies of the small and large intestine. In: Feldman M Scharschmidt BF, editors. Gastrointestinal and liver disease: pathophysiology, diagnosis, management. 6th edition. Philadelphia: WB Saunders; 1998. p. 1419–36.
9. Khan FA, Selvaggi G. Overview of intestinal and multivisceral transplantation. Available at: http://www.uptodate.com. Accessed October 21, 2009.
10. Park BK, De Angelis M. Intestine transplantation. In: Ohler L, Cupples SA, editors. Core curriculum for transplant nurses. St Louis: Mosby; 2008. p. 483–509.
11. Johnson R, Monkhouse S. Postoperative fluid and electrolyte balance: alarming audit results. J Perioper Pract 2009;19:291–4.
12. Ramsay MAE. Acute post operative pain management. BUMC Proc 2000;13:244–7.
13. Lisson EL. Ethical issues related to pain control. Nurs Clin North Am 1987;22:649–59.
14. Winslow E. Effective pain management. Am J Nurs 1998;7:16HH–16II.
15. Beck SL, Towsley GL, Berry PH, et al. Measuring the quality of care related to pain management. Nurs Res 2010;59(2):85–92.
16. Flaherty E. Using pain rating scales with older adults. Am J Nurs 2008;108(6);40–4.
17. Yagi M, Sakamoto K, Hasebe K, et al. Effect of a glutamine enriched diet on small bowel allograft during immunosuppressive therapy. Nutrition 1997;13(9):778–82.

18. Brook G. Quality of life issues: parenteral nutrition to small bowel transplantation: a review. Nutrition 1998;14(10):813–6.

19. Padula CA, Kenny A, Planchon C, et al. Enteral feeding: what the evidence says. Am J Nurs 2004;104(7):62–9.

20. Kenny DJ, Goodman P. Care of the patient with the enteral tube feeding. Nurs Res 2010;59(1S):S22–S31.

21. Serna ED, McCarthy M. Heads up to prevent aspiration during enteral feeding. Nursing 2006;36(1):76–7.

22. Boullata J. Drug administration through an enteral feeding tube. Am J Nurs 2009; 109(10):34–41.

23. Rolstad BS, Erwin-Toth PL. Peristomal skin complications: prevention and management. Ostomy Wound Manage 2004;50(9):68–77.

24. Lewis SM, Collier IC, Heilkemper MM. Ostomy care. In: Medical surgical nursing. 4th edition. St Louis: Mosby; 1996. p. 1228-9.

25. Wu T, Demitris AJ. Histopathology of intestinal transplantation. In: Langnas AN, Goulet O, Quigley EMM, et al, editors. Intestinal failure: diagnosis, management and transplantation. New York: Blackwell; 2008. p. 322–30.

26. de Bruin RWF, Stein-Oakley AN, Kouwenhoven EA, et al. Functional, histological and inflammatory changes in chronically rejecting small bowel transplants. Transpl Int 2000;13:1–11.

27. Abu-elmagd K, Bond G, Reyes J, et al. Intestinal transplantation: a coming of age. Adv Surg 2002;36:65–101.

28. Park BK. Intestine transplantation. Available at: http://www.medscape.com/viewarticle/436543. Accessed December 18, 2007.

29. Stitt NL. Infection in the transplant recipient: CMV. Medscape Nurses. Available at: http://www.medscape.com/viewarticle/451788. Accessed August 1, 2011.

30. Pascher A, Kohler S, Neuhaus P, et al. Present status and future perspectives of intestinal transplantation. Transpl Int 2008;21:401–14.

31. Allen U, Alfieri C, Preiksaitis J, et al. Epstein Barr virus infection in transplant recipients: summary of a workshop on surveillance, prevention and treatment. Can J Infect Dis 2002;13(2):89–99.

32. Mazariegos GV, Abu-Elmagd K, Jaffe R, et al. Graft versus host disease in intestinal transplantation. Am J Transplant 2004;4(9):1459–65.

33. Horslen SP. Optimal management of the post intestinal transplant patients. Gastroenterology 2006;130:S163–9.

34. Singh N. Fungal infections in the recipients of solid organ transplant. Infect Dis Clin North Am 2003;17(1):113–34.

35. Fungal infections. Am J Transplant 2004;4(Suppl 10):110–34.

36. Patterson TF. Approaches to fungal diagnosis in transplantation. Transplant Infect Dis 1999;1:262–72.

37. Fryer JP. Intestinal transplantation. In: Stuart FP, Abecassis MM, Kaufman DB, editors. Organ transplantation. Austin (TX): Landes Bioscience; 2000. p. 208–22. Available at: http://www.ncbi.nlm.nih.gov/pmc/articles/PMC1856585/?tool=pubmed-r4-13. Accessed August 3, 2011.

Heart Transplantation

Jeannine V. DiNella, RN, MSN[a],*, Jennifer Bowman, RN, BSN, MBA[b]

KEYWORDS

- Heart transplantation • Heart failure
- Ventricular assist device • End-stage heart disease

It has been over 40 years since the first human-to-human heart transplant was performed in Capetown, South Africa by Christiaan Barnard in December 1967.[1] At that time, survival was measured in terms of days or weeks.[1] Inadequate understanding of early postoperative complications as well as lack of tools to address the problems of acute rejection and opportunistic infection initially led to poor results.[2]

During the next two decades, refinement of donor and recipient selection methods, improved donor heart recovery and management, and the introduction of cyclosporine as the first main immunosuppressive agent significantly improved survival.[2] Today, heart transplantation is a viable treatment option for end-stage disease for patients of almost any age. Older patients are more often being considered as well as a greater proportion of younger patients who are born with complex congenital heart disease.[2] This has been made possible by ongoing research and the introduction of improved therapies. This article discusses the most current information related to taking care of heart transplant patients.

PATHOPHYSIOLOGY

The primary indication for adult heart transplantation during the last 5 years has gradually shifted from an equal split between coronary heart failure and noncoronary cardiomyopathy to a significantly greater proportion of patients with noncoronary cardiomyopathy: 50% versus 34% for January to June 2007.[3] Adult congenital heart disease (3%), retransplantation (2%), and valvular heart disease (2%) account for the remaining others.[3]

"Heart failure (HF) is a complex clinical syndrome that can result from any structural or functional cardiac disorder that impairs the ability of the ventricle to fill with or eject blood."[4] HF is an important cause of morbidity and mortality and is associated with high costs in care. A heart transplant may be recommended for patients with severe

The authors have nothing to disclose.

[a] UPMC Presbyterian, University of Pittsburgh Medical Center, Unit 9D 23.2, 200 Lothrop Street, Pittsburgh, PA 15213, USA

[b] Cardiothoracic Transplant Institute, UPMC Presbyterian, University of Pittsburgh Medical Center, 200 Lothrop Street, Pittsburgh, PA 15213, USA

* Corresponding author.

E-mail address: dinellaj@upmc.edu

doi:10.1016/j.ccell.2011.08.005
ccnursing.theclinics.com

HF, New York Heart Association Class III–IV, and when medications and surgery are no longer a feasible treatment alternative. Possible causes of severe HF are coronary artery disease, cardiomyopathy, and heart valve disease with congestive HF. Severe heart defects that are present at birth and cannot be corrected with surgery, and life-threatening abnormal heart beats or rhythms that do not respond to other therapy are also recommendations for transplant.[5]

HF caused by systolic dysfunction is more readily recognized. The ventricle cannot contract normally and pump sufficient blood. It is characterized by a decreased ejection fraction (<45%). The strength of ventricular contraction is inadequate for creating an adequate stroke volume, resulting in inadequate cardiac output. In diastolic dysfunction, the ventricle cannot relax and fill normally and has a stiffer ventricular wall. Therefore, there is inadequate stroke volume and there is an elevation in end-diastolic pressures.

WORKUP

Before the workup begins, the practitioner will treat the patient with routine exercise, sodium and fluid retention, a smoking cessation program if needed, and pharmacologic therapy. Patients with refractory HF may need to begin inotropic support. When these efforts fail, the practitioner will recommend that the patient send their clinical information to potential transplant centers. The purpose of the evaluation process is to determine the likelihood that the patient will meet criteria to be listed, and they will have the best chance of survival after the surgery.

Transplant centers will begin by reviewing all of the patient's information and order further testing. As part of the evaluation process, they will determine if the heart transplant candidate will be able to resume an active and normal lifestyle after surgery. Another very important component that is discussed among the transplant team is the patient's ability to comply with the strict guidelines that must be followed to maintain the allograft after the transplant.

Predictors of noncompliance can include inconsistency in taking medications, poor attendance at scheduled clinic appointments, excess drug and alcohol use, inadequate diet, and lack of family support. The transplant team attempts to be proactive and seek to identify all issues that could be problematic for the patient, such as inadequate coverage for immunosuppressant medications, inability to make follow-up appointments at the transplant center, lack of funding to pay for other costs needed to sustain the organ transplant such as travel costs to and from the transplant center, cost of day care if needed, co-pays for office visits, and lack of family support, to name a few.[6]

Social workers are involved in the selection process in an attempt to assess their home situation and finances. They also help the team in determining if the patient will be compliant with the follow-up care that is expected of them.

The team should also assess for HF severity, evaluate multiorgan function, infectious serology, vaccination history, malignancy history, and provide general consults such as psychiatry, financial, dental, nutritional, oncology, and social work.[7] Each patient undergoes numerous testing such as laboratory studies, electrocadiograms (ECG), echocardiograms, cardiac catheterizations, pulmonary function testing, and many more. These tests are performed not only because they are required, but also to diagnosis and treat any previously undiagnosed illnesses. Further along in the process, the patient undergoes tissue testing and blood typing to help ensure that the host will not reject the donated heart.[5]

After the required testing is complete, the transplant team decides if the patient is a candidate to be placed on the active list. Each center has its own policies and procedures regarding illnesses that put the patient in a higher risk category and therefore reject the candidate for listing. The major diagnosis that prevents a person from being eligible for cardiac transplantation is fixed pulmonary hypertension. Other indications include, but are not limited to, the following: advanced age, morbid obesity, active neoplasm, severe irreversible respiratory conditions, AIDS, current substance abuse, psychosocial instability, severe mental illness, and suicidal behavior.[8]

Once the team decides that they have a qualified recipient, accepted patients are listed on the United Network for Organ Sharing (UNOS). Patients are either listed as a 1A, 1B, or 2. Patients may move back and forth among these categories because of the delicate nature of their condition. Patients could remain on the list from days to several years.[8]

WAITING LIST

Patients on the waiting list for a donor heart receive ongoing treatment for HF and other medical conditions. In the United States, UNOS is contracted by the federal government to regulate donor heart allocation and has a priority system that is based on the severity of cardiac illness, geographic distance between donor and recipient, length of time on the waiting list, and ABO blood group compatibility. Based on the Organ Procurement and Transplant Network data as reported on April 23, 2010, there are approximately 3200 patients waiting for heart transplants in the United States.[9] The demand for organs greatly outweighs the supply, and consequently many patients die before transplant.

Many transplant centers now have other treatment options available to patients while they are waiting for an organ. Many centers will place an implantable defibrillator in patients before surgery. Another treatment that may be recommended to waiting list patients is an implanted mechanical pump called a ventricular assist device (VAD), which is known as a "bridge to transplant."

Risks of transplant include blood clots (deep venous thrombosis), damage to the kidneys, liver, or other body organs from anti-rejection (immunosuppression) medications, heart attack or stroke, heart rhythm problems, and increased risk for infections due to anti-rejection (immunosuppression) medications and wound infections.[5]

PROCEDURE

When the recipient arrives at the operating room (OR), hemodynamic monitoring lines are placed and operation of the cardiopulmonary bypass machine is initiated. There are two very different surgical techniques: the orthotopic approach and heterotopic transplantation.[10]

- **Orthotopic approach.** The more common of the two procedures, the orthotopic approach, requires replacing the recipient heart with the donor heart. After the donor heart is removed, preserved, and packed for transport, it must be transplanted into the recipient within 4 to 5 hours. The recipient receives general anesthesia and is placed on a bypass machine to oxygenate the blood while the heart transplant is being performed. After the recipient's heart is removed, the donor heart is prepared to fit and implantation begins.
- **Heterotopic approach.** Heterotopic transplantation, also called "piggyback" transplantation, is accomplished by leaving the recipient's heart in place and connecting the donor heart to the right side of the chest. The procedure is rare compared to orthotopic transplantation and is advantageous because the new heart can act as an assist device if complications occur.

PREPARING THE PATIENT FOR HEART TRANSPLANTATION SURGERY

There are many laboratory tests that must be completed including a blood type and crossmatch, especially for patients who might potentially need cytomegalovirus (CMV)-negative blood. A chest radiograph is to be completed and the physician may order an ECG. The recipient will be on hemodynamic monitoring and will receive nothing by mouth. The health care team ensures that the ICD is turned off. According to protocols in the facility, measurement of vital signs, weight, intake and output, consent forms, placement of IVs, and preoperative medications are to be completed. The patient will wait in the hospital until it is determined that the donor is a match for him or her. The patient could be waiting for many hours during this process while the donor tissue is being examined and tested for antibodies against the recipient. If it is determined that the patient is a match, he or she is taken to the operating room, and then sent to the cardiothoracic intensive care unit after the surgery. During this process, the donor information must not be revealed to the recipient, as this is strictly confidential information.

NURSING CARE

Early postoperative care of a heart transplant recipient remains a challenge, with approximately 12% of recipients not surviving the first 3 postoperative months, according to the Registry of the International Society for Heart & Lung Transplantation (ISHLT).[3] Goals of nursing care should include maintaining graft function and hemodynamic stability, ensuring proper ventilation and oxygenation, and prevention or early recognition of complications. The nurses will need to report trends when caring for their patients.

The patient arrives intubated and sedated with dressings intact that remain 24 to 48 hours, unless bleeding occurs that would necessitate removal of the dressing. There will be mediastinal pericardial drains and perhaps pleural drains.

Vital signs and hemodynamic monitoring will include blood pressure via the arterial line, pulmonary artery pressures, central venous pressure, cardiac output and index, SvO_2 (percentage of oxygen saturation in the pulmonary arterial blood), and pulse oximetry.

Hemodynamic compromise is defined as one or more of the following[11]:

- A reduction in cardiac output (<4.0 L/min) or cardiac index (<2.0 L/min per m^2)
- A decrease in pulmonary artery saturation ($<50\%$)
- An elevation in pulmonary artery or pulmonary capillary wedge pressure.

Denervation in heart transplantation means removing the organ's nerve supply, after which the transplanted heart lacks sympathetic and parasympathetic innervation. As a result in some cases, vasculopathy generally progresses silently and, in some cases, rapidly. Atropine will not be effective in bradycardia because the mechanism of action is to block input from the parasympathetic nerves; isoproterenol therefore may be used. The unique physiology has several effects[7]:

- Bradydysrhythmias may be observed in the immediate postoperative period; chronotropic support or pacing may be required.
- There may be a unique response to activity, exercise, and stressors.

Contractility, systolic function, and heart rate may be impaired and may necessitate inotropic or chronotropic support. If a patient has an increase in cardiac output, it may indicate sepsis. Low cardiac output may represent a decrease in contractility or left ventricular failure. If a patient's stroke volume is decreased, this can be HF related.

Certain intravenous medications may be needed. Telemetry monitoring is required and epicardial pacing may be needed. Nursing staff will be assessing for dysrhythmias that may indicate rejection and a pacer may be needed for atrial pacing or atrioventricular pacing. Monitoring of intake and output is required as well as pain management and laboratory tests.

The nurse must monitor blood gases to guide weaning from the ventilator. This typically begins 6 to 8 hours postoperatively. After extubation, aggressive pulmonary toileting is needed to decrease pneumonia and atelectasis. Neurologic status and drainage output must be monitored as well.

A prolonged stay in the intensive care unit may be necessary if the patient has complications such as bleeding, right-sided cardiac dysfunction, or biventricular failure requiring multiple inotrope therapy, an intra-aortic balloon pump or VAD.

COMPLICATIONS

From January 2002 to June 2006, the International Society for Heart & Lung Transplantation (2008) focused their analysis of 1-year mortality. Requiring short-term extracorporeal mechanical circulatory support, and having adult congenital heart disease as the indication for transplantation remained powerful risk factors for 1-year mortality, increasing the relative risk by two- to threefold. Despite the very high risk, it is important to note that these represent fewer than 2% and 3%, respectively, of the transplants performed during this time interval. Requiring dialysis or mechanical ventilation at the time of transplant each increased the risk of mortality by approximately 50%, yet represented only fewer than 3% of transplants. Treating an infection with intravenous antibiotics within 2 weeks before transplant increased the risk of mortality by 30%. Compatible but nonidentical ABO matching and prior blood transfusions were associated with 25% and 19% increases, respectively, in the risk of 1-year mortality. Coronary artery disease as the cause for end-stage HF was associated with a 16% greater risk for mortality compared with a cardiomyopathy indication.[15]

Complications can also arise from medications. Many of the drugs that are used are very powerful and can be toxic, especially to kidneys. Drugs such as tacrolimus and cyclosporin are nephrotoxic and frequent laboratory tests are needed to monitor patients for this possible effect. Patients can develop a plethora of side effects that are very specific for each medication. For the purpose of this article we do not discuss them in detail.

There are many complications that the health care team must monitor: bleeding, hypertension, infection, cardiac tamponade, pleural effusions, issues with cardiac output, dysrhythmias, fluid imbalances/hypovolemia, renal dysfunction, wound infections, hypo/hyperglycemia, alteration in bowel function, nutrition deficits, and self-care issues such as not wanting to participate in one's care.[8]

Significant risk factors impairing a continuous rather than categorical impact have remained relatively unchanged from past years and include recipient age, donor age, recipient height (inverse curvilinear), donor heart ischemic time, donor body mass index (inverse), transplant center volume (inverse), recipient pulmonary artery diastolic pressure, pretransplant recipient bilirubin level, and pretransplant recipient creatinine level. Preoperative use of a pulsatile ventricular assist device (VAD, long-term, chronic type) was associated with a 26% increase in mortality risk.[3]

REJECTION

Rejection is the process whereby the body's immune system attempts to destroy the allograft.[8] The current gold standard for recognizing rejection is the endomyocardial biopsy. Biopsies are performed more frequently during the first 6 to 12 months posttransplantation and vary depending on each center's protocol. This brief procedure is performed in the catheterization laboratory and is usually an outpatient procedure. It involves placing a catheter through the right internal jugular vein to obtain very tiny tissue samples that are examined for rejection. Sometimes the physician must enter through the groin because of the patient's anatomy. Once the samples are examined, the patient follows up with his or her physician in a few days for results. Depending on the results, the practitioner may increase the patient's medication (immunosuppressants and steroids) or the patient may be hospitalized for more involved therapy such as strong anti-rejection medications.[8] Some centers also use noninvasive testing through gene expression in blood samples and does not require the patient to have routine heart biopsies.

Rejection can be mediated by either cellular or humoral factors. Cellular rejection, the most common type, is mediated by T cells. Surface cell antigens of the allograft are recognized as foreign. Interleukins are produced that activate cytotoxic cells that in turn attempt to destroy the allograft. Humoral rejection acts differently in that platelet aggregation forms, which activates the clotting cascade. This causes reduced blood flow to the organs, which results in damage to the coronary arteries, hypotension, and shock.[8]

Each organ has its own method of identifying rejection. For heart transplantation, there are four categories: 0 R, no acute rejection; Grade 1 R, mild rejection; Grade 2 R, moderate rejection; and Grade 3 R, severe rejection.[3,12] If and when rejection is identified, the physician treats the patient per center protocol. Typically the first-line treatment is high-dose intravenous or oral steroid doses. It must be stressed that if rejection is identified, the patient needs to be watched closely to try to prevent further episodes. Heart transplant recipients typically have two to three episodes of acute rejection in the first year after transplantation, with a 50% to 80% chance of having at least one rejection episode, most commonly in the first 6 months.[12]

Symptoms of rejection may include but are not limited to signs of left ventricular dysfunction such as dyspnea, syncope, and jugular venous distention, generalized flulike infection, shortness of breath, low-grade fever, edema, and general fatigue. Acute rejection is more serious and the patient may present with a variety of tachyarrhythmias, atrial more often than ventricular.[5,11]

Beyond the first year, transplant vasculopathy (also called transplant coronary artery disease or cardiac allograft vasculopathy) is the second most common cause of death, after malignancy.[12] Transplant vasculopathy typically progresses; however, occasional patients progress rapidly and unpredictably.[12] Cardiac transplant recipients have afferently as well as efferently denervated hearts; although there is evidence for reinnervation in some patients by 5 years after transplantation, the degree of reinnervation is generally incomplete.[7,12] As a result, patients with transplant vasculopathy seldom experience the classic symptom of angina pectoris.

Silent myocardial infarction, sudden death, and progressive HF are common presentations of transplant vasculopathy. Symptoms associated with exertion, such as dyspnea, diaphoresis, gastrointestinal distress, presyncope, or syncope, are often infrequent, atypical, and may be misleading.[7,12]

The diagnosis is established by angiography. Although coronary angiography is the gold standard for the diagnosis of nontransplant atherosclerosis, it is less sensitive in detecting transplant vasculopathy. This is due to the often diffuse and concentric nature of this disease, as opposed to the focal and eccentric pattern of nontransplant atherosclerosis.[7,12] Intravascular (intracoronary) ultrasound (IVUS) has been used because it is possible to visualize these layers and thereby detect abnormal thickening of the intima.

DISCHARGE

The recovery period is approximately 6 months. The patient will be assigned to a heart transplant coordinator and a cardiologist who will follow him or her until death. The coordinator assists in finding a facility to begin cardiac rehabilitation. Weekly blood work is required to observe immunosppression levels, infection, kidney function, liver function, CMV infection, lipids, and nutrition status. Once the patient's labs become stable, he or she will eventually require laboratory tests only on a monthly basis. Biopsies of the heart muscle are often performed every month during the first 6 to 12 months after transplant, and then only as indicated. Some centers use gene expression diagnostics through blood sampling.

The goal of immunosuppression therapy is to prevent/treat rejection while minimizing the risk of infection or cancer. Sometimes a patient will have induction therapy, which is a more concentrated immunosuppression in the early days after transplantation. The justification for this is to provide intensive immunosuppression at the time when alloimmune response is most intense.[2] Maintenance immunosuppression is to achieve host–graft adaptation while minimizing the risk of infection or cancer.[2] Tacrolimus is favored in the presence of higher risk of rejection, preexisting hypertension, or hyperlipidemia, whereas cyclosporin is favored in the presence of diabetes mellitus.[2]

It is important that each patient have a primary care physician (PCP) or general practitioner who can ensure that all other routine examinations such as mammograms, prostrate exams, eye exams, and similar tests are performed. Because most patients do not live in close proximity to their transplant facility, it is important to have a physician who can assess them quickly if needed. It is vital to teach heart transplant recipients when they need to contact their transplant center versus their PCP. Patients should contact their transplant coordinator for a fever of 38.5°C or higher, blood pressure readings that are higher than usual, red or rusty-brown colored urine, burning with urination, edema in the face, abdomen, or feet, weight gain of 2 to 3 pounds overnight, pain, productive cough, dizziness, constant nausea or vomiting, and a change in bowel habits. Patients should contact their PCP for any other issues not related to their transplant. Treatment for many of these symptoms can be communicated over the telephone per each center's protocol without sending the patient to an emergency room.

Patients should also be assigned a registered dietitian. The dietician develops nutrition therapy for patients before and after transplantation. Dieticians educate patients about maintaining weight and minimizing side effects of anti-rejection drug therapy.

All organ transplant patients are at risk of developing skin cancer because of the anti-rejection medications. Malignancies represent the leading cause of death among long-term survivors and equal cardiac allograft vasculopathy as a cause of death in recipients who live longer than 5 years.[8] Important practices to teach patients are the following: always use sunscreen on all exposed skin areas, wear sunglasses, hats, and protective clothing, and make an annual appointment with a dermatologist to assess for any signs of skin cancer.

Patients need to be taught preventative measures to help avoid developing the disease such as smoking cessation, avoiding alcohol, eating a well-balanced diet rich in calcium and vitamin D, possibly taking calcium plus vitamin D supplements, and engaging in weight-bearing exercise. Another necessary subject to discuss with patients is bone density screening test at least every 2 years. Heart and all other transplant patients must take prednisone to protect the allograft. Unfortunately, prednisone has many unwanted side effects such weight gain, acne, moodiness, and osteoporosis.

There is much to learn with regard to a heart transplant. Patients are given printed material upon discharge that contains a mountain of information. It is so essential for patients to try to read the material, learn their medications, and schedule appointments. Many patients become confused and frustrated, and for this reason it is crucial for them to contact their coordinator for any questions they may have. Each patient's recovery time is different and depends on factors such as his or her age and disease process before transplant. It is very important to encourage patients and teach them how to cope with their new organ.

SURVIVAL

As of June 5, 2009, the 1-year survival rate was 88.0% for males and 77.2% for females; the 3-year survival rate was approximately 79.3% for males and 77.2% for females. The 5-year survival rate was 73.1% for males and 67.4% for females.[13] Heart transplant has limited long-term survival; therefore, some recipients are considered candidates for retransplantation. In 2007, a report from ISHLT registry for the most recent cohort transplanted between January 1, 2004 to June 30, 2006, 3% of reported cases were retransplants.[9] Patients undergoing retransplantation between 2002 and 2005 experienced a 1-year survival rate of approximately 85%.[9]

SUMMARY

Cardiac transplantation remains a life-prolonging process. Survival after heart transplantation has improved despite a sicker incoming patient population. The field of heart transplantation is constantly evolving. Advances in organ preservation, immune monitoring, and improved immunosuppressive regimens will continue to develop over time. The impact of the newest immunosuppressive agents and protocols, improved diagnostic testing, and new management strategies is yet to be determined.[3] The potential of cell therapy is still under evaluation and the field is still in its infancy but rapidly evolving; the key to the future in this field may not be the delivery of the cells themselves but understanding how they interact with one another at a molecular level and, in particular, with resident stem cells in cardiac tissue.[14] In addition to the medical advances, health care professionals need to educate the public about the benefits of transplantation as well.

REFERENCES

1. Hunt SA. Taking heart — cardiac transplantation past, present, and future. N Engl J Med 2006;355:231–5.
2. Hunt SA, Haddad F. The changing face of heart transplantation. Am Coll Cardiol 2008;52(8):587–98.
3. Taylor DO, Edwards LB, Aurora P, et al. Registry of the International Society of Heart and Lung Transplantation: twenty-fifth official adult heart transplant report–2008. J Heart Lung Transplant 2008;27:943–56.
4. Hunt SA, Abraham WT, Chin MH, et al. 2009 focused update incorporated into the ACC/AHA 2005 Guidelines for the Diagnosis and Management of Heart Failure in Adults: a report of the American College of Cardiology Foundation/American Heart Association Task Force on Practice Guidelines developed in collaboration with the International Society for Heart and Lung Transplantation. J Am Coll Cardiol 2009; 53(15):e7.

5. Lee J. Heart transplant. Available at: http://www.nlm.nih.gov/medlineplus/ency/article/003003.htm. Accessed May 3, 2010.

6. Sherry DC, Simmons B, Wung SF, et al. Noncompliance in heart transplantation: a role for the advanced practice nurse. Prog Cardiovasc Nurs 2003;18(3):141–6.

7. Hartley C, Fisher G, Cupples S. In: Ohler L, Cupples S, editors. Core curriculum for transplant nurses. Philadelphia: Mosby/Elsevier; 2008. p. 322–3.

8. Cupples SA, Ohler L, editors. Transplantation nursing secrets. Philadelphia: Hanley & Belfus; 2003. p. 85–105.

9. Organ Procurement and Transplant Network. Available at: www.optn.org. Accessed May 3, 2010.

10. United Network for Organ Sharing. Available at: http://www.transplantliving.org/duringthetransplant/heart.aspx. Accessed May 3, 2010.

11. Miller BW. Solid organ transplant medicine. In: Cooper DH, Kraniak AJ, Lubner SJ, et al, editors. The Washington manual of medical therapeutics. 32nd edition. St. Louis (MO): Kluwer/Lippincott Williams & Wilkins; 2007. p. 433.

12. Eisen HJ, Ross H. Natural history and diagnosis of cardiac transplant vasculopathy; Up to Date. Available at: http://www.uptodate.com/online/content/topic.do?topicKey=hrt_tran/4889&selectedTitle=1%7E150&source=search_result. Accessed March 26, 2010.

13. Heart transplant statistics. Available at: http://www.americanheart.org/presenter.pjhtml?identifier=4588. Accessed May 3, 2010.

14. Boilson BA, Raichlin E, Park SJ, et al. Device therapy and cardiac transplantation for end-stage heart failure. Curr Probl Cardiol 2010;35(1):8–64.

15. International Society for Heart & Lung Transplantation. Available at: http://www.ishlt.org/registries/slides.asp?slides=heartLungRegistry&year=2008. Accessed May 3, 2010.

Lung Transplant

Elisabeth L. George, RN, PhD[a],*,
Jane Guttendorf, RN, MSN, CRNP, ACNP-BC[b]

KEYWORDS

- Lung transplantation • Critically ill • Intensive care
- Critical care nurse

OVERVIEW

History

The modern era of transplantation began in the 1980s with the introduction of cyclosporine.[1] Current volume statistics indicate that lung transplantation is a recognized option for select patients with end-stage lung disease. Based on Organ Procurement and Transplant Network data as of April 16, 2010, 19,907 patients have undergone isolated lung transplant and 1027 patients have undergone heart-lung procedures. Because of advancements in immunosuppression, surgical techniques, donor selection and criteria, and preoperative and postoperative patient management, there has been marked improvement in outcomes since the 1990s. Based on current data, the overall adjusted 1-year survival rate is 86% and the adjusted 5-year survival is 56% (adjusted death rates factor in recipient, donor, and transplant risks).[2] It is important to note that patient survival varies depending on many factors including but not limited to: the primary lung disease, procedure type, recipient comorbidities, age of recipient, characteristics of the donor lungs, and, more recently, on changes in allocation of available organs to those with the greater likelihood of survival.[2,3]

Experience since the first lung transplant by James Hardy over 40 years ago has resulted in substantial improvements in outcomes, yet lung transplant recipients do not experience the same long-term outcomes as other solid organ recipients.[4] Common limiting factors to successful transplantation include available donor organs, rejection, infection, and organ system dysfunction. Additional factors impacting outcomes for lung transplant recipients include early issues with preservation injury and later bronchiolitis obliterans syndrome (BOS) resulting in chronic rejection. Chronic rejection impacts both the quality of life (QOL) and long-term survival rates.

[a] Advanced Practice Nurse Critical Care, Department of Nursing, University of Pittsburgh Medical Center–Presbyterian Shadyside, 200 Lothrop Street, Pittsburgh, PA 15213, USA
[b] Cardiothoracic ICU, Department of Critical Care Medicine, University of Pittsburgh Medical Center–Presbyterian Shadyside, 200 Lothrop Street, Pittsburgh, PA 15213, USA
* Corresponding author.
E-mail address: georgebl@upmc.edu

Crit Care Nurs Clin N Am 23 (2011) 481–503
doi:10.1016/j.ccell.2011.06.002
0899-5885/11/$ – see front matter © 2011 Published by Elsevier Inc.

Indication

Indications for lung transplant continue to evolve. Transplantation is indicated when other therapeutic options fail to produce improvement for patients with end-stage lung disease and the predicted life expectancy is less than 24 months. Timing for patient referral to transplant is key to the likelihood the patient will reach transplantation. Ideal timing is when patients have either or both a less than 50% two- to three-year predicted survival and a New York Heart Association class III or IV level of function.[5] Regardless, the mortality rate for patients waiting for lung transplantation in 2007 was about 13%.[6] The wait list mortality may be impacted by programs that list patients with high acuity and the increased number of recipients in the ICU at the time of transplant (9% increase in 2007).[2]

The initial recipient selection criteria developed in 1998 have been reconsidered related to evolving practices.[7] The revised criteria for recommended selection and contraindications are based on a consensus report and are adopted by The International Society for Heart and Lung Transplantation (ISHLT).[5] The general and relative contraindications are listed in detail in the International Guidelines for the Selection of Lung Transplant Candidates.[5] Absolute contraindications include: 1) malignancy in the last 2 years (with certain exceptions); 2) untreatable advanced dysfunction of another organ system; 3) chronic extra pulmonary infection that is noncurable including chronic active viral hepatitis B, hepatitis C, and human immunodeficiency virus; 4) significant chest wall/spinal deformity; 5) documented nonadherence to medical therapy; 6) untreatable psychiatric or psychological conditions; 7) lack of consistent social support; and 8) substance addiction that is active or within the last 6 months. Relative contraindications include: 1) age older than 65 years; 2) critical or unstable clinical conditions; 3) severely limited functional status with limited rehabilitation potential; 4) colonization with highly resistant or highly virulent bacteria, mycobacterium, or fungi; 5) severe obesity (body mass index greater than 30 kg/m; 6) severe or symptomatic osteoporosis; 7) mechanical ventilation (MV); and 8) other medical conditions that have not resulted in end-stage disease (should be treated pretransplantation). Recommendations for patient referral focus on specific diagnostic criteria for various lung diseases.[8]

There is limited prospective randomized research to support the current recommendations, which result in variation in practice. It is well known that candidate selection differs between centers, and candidates declined at one center can often be accepted at another center.[9] Variance in applying selection criteria for age limits, procedure of choice, surgical technique, colonized or infected patients, and body size are noted in the literature with good outcomes. This extension of the criteria is thought to be contributing to a more critically ill population of recipients and the impact on outcomes is being evaluated. For example, the percentage of lung transplants in patients greater than 65 years of age has been increasing. One center found no difference in 1-year and 3-year survival rates in a group 65 years of age or older compared with a similar group under age 65.[10] In comparison, in 2006 the highest death rates were for those aged 65 or older.[2] Mechanical ventilation pretransplant is considered a risk factor, but one study demonstrated similar 1-year survival rates between those on MV pretransplant and those not on MV.[11]

Choice of Procedure

Current procedural options include single lung transplantation (SLT), bilateral sequential or double-lung transplantation (BLT), heart-lung transplantation (HLT), and living donor lobar lung transplantation. In the earlier era, the thought was to maximize the

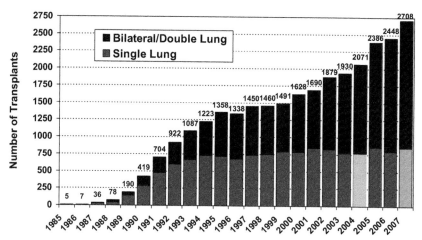

Fig. 1. This figure shows the number of lung transplants that were reported to the ISHLT Transplant Registry for the years 1985 to 2007. (This may not be reflective of all centers worldwide performing lung transplants.) Note the relative increase in the number of bilateral/double lung procedures relative to the stable number of single lung transplant procedures performed over the range of years. (With permission from The International Society of Heart & Lung Transplantation. Add J Heart Lung Transplant 2009;28:989–1049.)

benefit of a limited donor source to increase the number of recipients, thereby favoring the choice to perform single lung transplants. Heart-lung procedures were reserved for patients with end-stage lung disease combined with an irreparable heart defect. Double lung procedures were indicated for patients with septic disease, and single lung procedures were considered for other end-stage lung diseases. Current trends favor more BLT for patients with pulmonary hypertension and even emphysema, which may reflect a bias that this procedure delays development of BOS.[12] In addition, bilateral recipients have a slight increase in median survival over SLT (5.9 vs 4.4 years, respectively).[13] Thus, BLT has been increasing, whereas the number of SLT is decreasing (**Fig. 1**).

Currently, the decision for which lung transplant procedure to perform is guided by the primary lung disease and the choice of the transplant center.[14] Either SLT or BLT is performed for chronic obstructive pulmonary disease, idiopathic interstitial pneumonias, and pulmonary hypertension depending on the center. Bilateral lung transplantation remains the procedure of choice for patients with cystic fibrosis related to the risk of infection. There is no clear preference for SLT or BLT for patients who develop secondary pulmonary hypertension. A heart-lung procedure is reserved for patients with end-stage lung disease and both right and left heart failure.

DONOR AND RECIPIENT SELECTION
Donor Selection

Lung transplantation remains limited by available donor organs, which impacts both waiting time for listed patients and thus the risk of dying before transplantation.[15] Numerous strategies to increase donor numbers have been tried such as living-donor lobar transplantation, non-heart–beating donors, and expansion of the selection criteria.[6] There are limited data regarding the specifics of human lung donors. A consensus report from The Pulmonary Council of ISHLT reviewed parameters of lung transplant donor acceptability.[16] The current recommendations for "ideal" lung donors include age less than 55 years, clear chest radiograph, ABO blood type compatibility, PaO_2 greater than 300 mm Hg on 100% FiO_2, minimal smoking history (<20 pack-years), no chest trauma, no evidence of aspiration/sepsis, no prior cardiopulmonary surgery, negative Gram stain of pulmonary secretions, and no purulent secretions with bronchoscopy.[16] Body size match between donor and recipient also has implications. Similar to extending the criteria for selection of lung transplant candidates, many centers have extended the general criteria for donors. The ultimate decision is most often individualized based on donor and recipient characteristics. The use of expanded criteria over the years has led to an increased use of donors who would have otherwise been refused. Nevertheless, there remains a need to define the limits of acceptance for donor lungs based on evidence.

The critical care nurse (CCN) plays an active role in identifying and often managing potential lung donors. Local organ procurement agencies should be notified according to institutional and state regulations to facilitate the donor process. The donor requires complex critical care management to maintain physiological stability and avoid organ failure.[17]

Allocation of Donor Lungs

It is important to note that the trends in lung and heart-lung transplantation in the United States have been impacted by the implementation of the Lung Allocation Scoring System (LAS) in May 2005.[18] Specific data comparisons of the "pre-LAS era" and "post-LAS era" have been addressed.[2] The intent of developing the LAS was to balance urgency with patient outcome and create a prioritization for patients with a high predicted survival benefit and short predicted waiting period survival. In comparison with the pre-LAS waiting list system, which was predominantly "time on the list," the LAS has resulted in a reduction of time on the waiting list, number of adults on the waiting list, and waiting list mortality.[2] Regardless, there is still a need for ongoing refinement in the calculation of the LAS score. For example, the current LAS does include QOL in the measure of posttransplant benefit.

Recipient Evaluation and Selection

Once the patient is referred to a transplant center, medical information is reviewed before a scheduled visit to rule out any contraindications to transplant. To ensure that the individual is an appropriate candidate, a multidisciplinary outpatient evaluation at the transplant center includes various tests and procedures of objective measures of disease as well as assessment for cognitive function, social supports, and other factors that may impact compliance with the postoperative regimen.[9] An example laboratory and diagnostic testing schedule for recipient evaluation from our institution is attached (see **Table 1**). Often, patients are referred to a transplant center not for immediate listing but for the process to be initiated (ie, patients with idiopathic pulmonary fibrosis) so that any contraindications to transplant can be managed. Preoperative considerations and management are impacted by patient diagnosis. Because time accrued is not a factor with current candidate listing, patients are usually not listed until they are in need of transplantation. Both candidates who are accepted for transplant and those who are not require comprehensive support because of the stress, anxiety, and fears that surround this process. At this time, education for those accepted to transplantation is usually initiated, such as social work assistance for support and insurance concerns. In addition, the LAS is assigned based on medical severity. Coordinators at transplant centers maintain close contact

Table 1
Example of lung transplant evaluation and diagnostic testing before recipient selection

Laboratory Testing	Radiology Testing	Diagnostic Testing	Consultant Evaluations
Blood type and screen (ABO)	Chest radiograph	Pulmonary function testing including lung volumes, DLCO, and ABG	Pulmonary Transplant team
Quick PRA	High-resolution CT scan of chest	Six-minute walk test	Cardiothoracic surgery transplant team
HLA tissue typing	Abdomen ultrasound	V/Q scan	Cardiology/Heart failure team
Urinalysis	Barium swallow	Esophageal manometry with pH probe	Social services
CBC with differential	Bone density scan	Peripheral arterial Dopplers of lower and upper extremities	Financial services
Platelets, PT, PTT		Carotid arterial Dopplers	Nutrition
Electrolytes, BUN, creatinine, glucose		EKG	Renal medicine
Twenty-four hour urine collection for creatinine clearance		Transthoracic echocardiogram	Endocrinology
Liver function studies		Myocardial perfusion imaging study	Rheumatology
Fasting lipid profile		Right heart catheterization	Psychiatry
BNP		Left heart catheterization	
PSA		Coronary angiography	
RPR		Flexible sigmoidoscopy	
HIV ELISA			
Hepatitis A, B, and C panels			
IgG serologies for CMV, EBV, HSV I and II, Varicella, and Toxoplasma			

Abbreviations: ABG, arterial blood gas; BNP, B-type natriuretic peptide; BUN, blood urea nitrogen; CBC, complete blood count; CT, computed tomography; DLCO, diffusion capacity; EKG, electrocardiogram; ELISA, enzyme-linked immunosorbent assay; IgG, immunoglobulin G; PRA, panel reactive antibody; PT, prothrombin time; PTT, partial thromboplastin time; PSA, prostate-specific antigen, RPR, rapid plasma reagin; V/Q, ventilation perfusion.
Adapted from University of Pittsburgh Presbyterian preoperative orders ©UPMC 2009.

with candidates to monitor health status, and some may require the candidate to relocate within a 2-hour drive of the transplant center.

OPERATIVE PROCEDURE

Standard monitoring is used for both SLT and BLT such as a pulmonary artery catheter, radial/femoral arterial lines, and urinary catheter.[15] A double lumen endotracheal intubation is routine to facilitate single lung ventilation during surgery. Transesophageal echo monitoring is used to monitor heart function and to evaluate the pulmonary vein anastomoses. Most adult lung transplants do not routinely require cardiopulmonary bypass (CPB), because this is reserved for patients with severe pulmonary hypertension or patients with cystic fibrosis who cannot tolerate one-lung ventilation. CPB may also be necessary if a heart procedure is also planned. Efforts are made to avoid bypass if possible because it increases the risk of bleeding.

For SLT, the side with the poorest ventilation and perfusion is selected for transplant.[15] BLT involves bilateral thoracotomies or the trans-sternal bilateral thoracotomy ("clamshell"). The standard approach to thoracotomy is usually a posterolateral thoracotomy incision, but some centers now use a smaller anterior axillary thoracotomy, either unilaterally or bilaterally.[19] Lung explantation and replacement focus on the integrity of the 3 main anastomoses: bronchus, pulmonary artery, and left atrium (pulmonary veins). Before closure, suture lines are checked for hemostasis and a bronchoscopy is performed to assess the bronchial anastomosis.[15] To limit the need for CBP, the least functioning lung is replaced first. It is ideal to remove adhesions before the lung is explanted to reduce the incidence of reperfusion edema.[15]

POSTOPERATIVE CARE

CCNs have noted the changing population of lung transplant recipients for whom they provide care. The current population of patients differs from earlier years as a result of expanded recipient selection such as the increase in age of recipients, as well as the expanded donor criteria. Also, as noted previously, an increased number of candidates are in the critical care units preoperatively, which suggests an increased acuity of patients presenting for transplant. The CCN must be able to constantly integrate the ongoing advancements in the field of lung transplantation with established nursing care standards.

The postoperative care of the lung transplant recipient is impacted by the patient's primary diagnosis, preoperative conditioning, and the type of procedure performed. In addition, the anatomy and physiology in the transplanted lung are altered and the degree of alteration is dependent on whether SLT, BLT, or HLT is performed. It is important for the nurse to recognize the impact of these changes on routine postoperative care.

Physiological and Anatomical Alterations Affecting Postoperative Care

The pulmonary system is disrupted by the removal of the diseased lung and the reimplantation of the allograft. Nerves (vagus and sympathetic), blood supply (pulmonary and brachial), and the lymphatic system are interrupted, which all impact nursing care.

Loss of innervation

The lung is without innervation below the level of the bronchial anastomosis. This impacts airway clearance because of absence of the cough reflex. The cough reflex is functional in the remaining lung if SLT was performed and also in the airways proximal to the airway anastomosis for both SLT and BLT.[20] Additionally, the normal ciliary transport of mucous is decreased and secretion clearance is reduced.[21] These changes require astute attention to postoperative airway clearance interventions such as suctioning and have implications for the development of respiratory infection and/or aspiration.

Airway hyperreactivity
Airway hyperreactivity (as assessed by aerosol challenge tests) is documented in lung and HLT transplant patients. This was initially not thought to have a major impact clinically, although attention to patient response is important during aerosol breathing treatments or other broncho-stimulating interventions. Data have indicated a link between metacholine challenge test responsiveness with the subsequent development of BOS.[22]

Control of ventilation
In the immediate postoperative period, control of ventilation is altered somewhat and the patient response to hypercapnia varies. In post-lung transplant chronic obstructive pulmonary disease recipients, a continuation of a blunted response to CO_2 levels was documented, but this was usually resolved within 3 weeks.[23]

Diffusion capacity and ventilation/perfusion (V/Q) changes postoperatively are dependent on the primary lung disease and the type of procedure performed. Diffusion improvement is greater in patients with emphysema versus those with interstitial lung disease receiving SLT.[24] After SLT, for patients with emphysema, ventilation usually favors the compliant native lung and about 50% to 80% of perfusion goes to allograft.[25,26] In patients with fibrosis or interstitial lung disease, both ventilation and perfusion are increased to the allograft because of high vascular resistance in the native lung.[27] Because of these physiological changes, the SLT recipient with pulmonary hypertension may be nearly completely dependent on the allograft for oxygenation and ventilation, in the early postoperative period. This becomes more of a concern for V/Q mismatch if there is any degree of allograft injury. In contrast, if there is injury to the allograft of an SLT with emphysema, the degree of V/Q mismatch and gas exchange abnormality is not as severe, because the more compliant native lung may play a greater role in gas exchange. These alternations in V/Q affect postoperative ventilator management and nursing care to optimize oxygenation.

Lymphatic disruption
The lung allograft is prone to dysfunction related to the loss of endothelial integrity from ischemia and the decrease in interstitial fluid clearance from lymphatic disruption. The impaired lymphatic drainage is a concern in the immediate postoperative period but does not seem as relevant in the long term as experimental data suggest that lymphatics return to function 3 to 6 weeks postoperatively.[27] In the early postoperative period these changes have implications for oxygenation and ventilation support.

Airway ischemia
Bronchial ischemia has an impact on the postoperative recovery. The bronchial arteries supplying the distal trachea, carina, and bronchi are severed during the lung transplant procedure and not reattached.[28] The resultant airway ischemia impacts the healing of the bronchial anastomosis and may result in dehiscence, stenosis, or

airway infections. Collateral blood supply from the pulmonary artery can develop, but may take weeks to months to form.[29] Currently, anastomotic complications are infrequent because of improvements in lung preservation, surgical technique, and early patient management. If dehiscence and necrosis occur, they can usually be managed by airway debridement.[15] Bronchial revascularization is not routinely performed, because it is technically challenging.[30] Some work has indicated that direct bronchial revascularization may postpone the developed of BOS.[31]

Diaphragm paralysis

Diaphragm paralysis from phrenic nerve damage is reported to occur in 3% to 30% of patients, which impacts the ability to wean from the ventilator postoperatively.[32] In chronic obstructive pulmonary disease recipients, diaphragmatic strength actually improves probably because of decreased lung volumes and the change in diaphragm configuration to a more normal shape.[33]

Swallowing dysfunction, aspiration, and gastric reflux

Injury to the vagus and recurrent laryngeal and superior laryngeal nerves during surgery may contribute to the incidence of oropharyngeal or gastric disorders. This combination of dysfunction may increase the risk for reflux, aspiration, and chronic bacterial airway colonization in the postoperative period.

The ability to swallow properly in the postoperative period has been receiving increased attention. One report indicates that over 70% of lung transplant recipients had abnormal swallow studies.[34] Local injury from endotracheal intubation can also contribute to this dysfunction. The increased risk for tracheal aspiration combined with impaired cough mechanisms creates a major concern for nursing care.

Because gastroesophageal reflux is common in patients with end-stage lung disease before transplant, many centers now screen for this disorder preoperatively and closely evaluate swallowing function. In addition, worsening of gastroesophageal dysfunction and delayed gastric emptying have been documented after lung transplant.[35]

Pulmonary Management

Early pulmonary care focuses on ventilator management, secretion clearance, monitoring for ischemic reperfusion injury (IRI) (primary graft dysfunction), and targeted early extubation.

Ventilator management

Inspired oxygen concentration is minimized to avoid injury from oxygen-free radicals, targeting oxygen titration to achieve PaO_2 of 70 to 90 mm Hg and oxygen saturations of 94% or greater. It is common for patients to arrive in the ICU from the operating room with oxygen concentrations (FiO_2) of 30% to 40%. An early chest radiograph may give an indication of baseline graft dysfunction (IRI); however, the radiographic appearance of graft dysfunction (diffuse pulmonary infiltrates) may worsen within the first 12 to 24 hours postoperatively. Other ventilator management strategies include moderate levels of positive end expiratory pressure (PEEP) to manage the hypoxemia, and diffuse capillary leak associated with pulmonary edema, a common manifestation of reperfusion injury/primary graft dysfunction.[9,36] Typically, patients with more severe reperfusion injury will require higher levels of PEEP and longer ventilator support. Lung protective strategies are used with target tidal volumes of 6 mL/kg ideal body weight, and peak inspiratory pressure and plateau pressure targets of less than 30 cm H_2O. Pressure-limited modes of ventilation may be required in patients with stiff, noncompliant lungs, generating high inspiratory airway pressures related to reperfusion injury. In rare instances when lung physiology is significantly discrepant between the right and left lungs (as may occur in a single lung recipient with a compliant emphysematous native lung and a stiff, noncompliant lung allograft), with evidence of cardiopulmonary compromise, independent or differential lung ventilation may be required.[15] This is accomplished via placement of a double lumen endobronchial tube, usually directed into the left mainstem bronchus, with placement confirmed bronchoscopically, and then use of 2 ventilators with different settings to achieve ventilatory goals for each of the respective lungs.

Secretion clearance

Secretion clearance is important to achieve successful extubation. If ischemic airway injury is significant, there may be sloughing of tissue into the airways, and this, coupled with secretion production, inadequate ciliary clearance, and ineffective cough, may impair airway clearance. Aggressive maneuvers to assist airway clearance are important, including early mobilization, pain management, and adequate suctioning. There is a low threshold for therapeutic bronchoscopy for evaluation of airway injury and to assist in clearance of secretions.

Early extubation

Early extubation is the goal when patients are able to oxygenate adequately with minimal inspired oxygen and low levels of PEEP (5 cm or less). Pain management is important to facilitate effective coughing and deep breathing. Patients with minimal IRI can be successfully weaned from MV and extubated within the first 8 to 12 hours. If moderate or severe IRI is present, patients may require more prolonged positive pressure ventilation before successful weaning and extubation can be achieved.

Failure to wean

Failure to wean from the ventilator may be due to fluid overload or positive fluid balance, because the transplanted lungs with impaired lymphatic drainage are sensitive to even mild fluid overload. Other contributing factors may include pain, deconditioning, inadequate secretion clearance, or, less likely, early infection (pneumonia) or diaphragmatic dysfunction. Although hypoxemia is the primary reason for respiratory failure in the early postoperative period, hypercapnia may be the reason for initial failure to wean or may be a cause of respiratory failure requiring reintubation, particularly in patients with preexisting carbon dioxide retention such as end-stage cystic fibrosis or chronic obstructive pulmonary disease.

Pleural drainage

Most patients have 2 to 3 chest drains on each operative side. Chest tubes placed anteriorly and directed apically will drain any air that accumulates. Tubes directed posteriorly and toward the lung base will drain any accumulated fluids or blood. Initially, drains are placed to suction and continue on suction until air leaks are no longer present. Apical tubes are usually removed first, once air leaks are resolved, and there is no evidence of pneumothorax on chest radiograph. Posterior or basilar drains are usually kept in place until drainage is minimal (<150 mL/d/tube) because it is difficult for patients to reabsorb residual pleural fluid without functioning lymphatic drainage. Persistent high volume pleural drainage should prompt evaluation for chylothorax, particularly if drainage increases after tube feedings or dietary intake are initiated or if fluid appears milky or cloudy.

Cardiovascular Management

After lung transplant, patients have continuous monitoring of electrocardiogram, arterial pressure, and oxygen saturation, as well as monitoring of pulmonary artery pressures, central venous pressure, and measurements of cardiac output and cardiac index (CI).

Management of hemodynamics

Postoperative hypertension should be managed aggressively because of risk of bleeding from vascular anastamoses (pulmonary artery, left atrium). Typically this can be managed with easily titratable medications such as nitroprusside, nitroglycerine, or nicardipine. Hypotension may be related to hypovolemia, vasodilation, or low CI, and is treated based on evaluation of filling pressures, CI, assessment of peripheral perfusion and urine output, assessment of the patient's ability to tolerate volume resuscitation relative to oxygenation, appearance of the chest radiograph, and ventilator requirements. Fluids are administered cautiously because the overriding goal is to maintain negative fluid balance. Fluids may be needed for managing hypotension or low CI associated with low filling pressures, or for low urine output associated with low filling pressures. Low CI is managed with volume if associated with low filling pressures or by the addition of inotropic agents. Findings from the intraoperative transesophageal echocardiogram can be helpful in identifying patients with underlying right or left ventricular dysfunction. Even in the absence of ventricular dysfunction intraoperatively, postoperative hemodynamics may warrant inotropic support, particularly in patients with changing pulmonary vascular resistance, recovery from CPB (if used), or ongoing bleeding or hypotension. Persistent hypotension in the setting of adequate CI can be managed with vasopressors.

Arrhythmia management

Common postoperative arrhythmias include atrial fibrillation, atrial flutter, and other supraventricular arrhythmias. In one series of patients, there was a 19% incidence of atrial fibrillation or atrial flutter after BLT similar to that of their postoperative coronary artery bypass graft surgery patients.[37] This occurred in spite of the pulmonary vein isolation that occurs during anastamosis of the donor right and left pulmonary veins via atrial cuffs to the posterior left atrial wall of the recipient and was not related to increased left atrial size.[37] Management options may be limited by concomitant use of vasopressor or inotropic agents, considerations for drug-drug interactions between antiarrhythmic agents and common immunosuppressant agents, and side effect profiles of certain antiarrhythmic agents in patients undergoing lung transplants. Although commonly used to control rate and attempt conversion of atrial fibrillation in other patients undergoing cardiothoracic surgery, amiodarone (Cordarone) may be less useful in long-term management of atrial arrhythmias in patients with lung transplants because of the potential for pulmonary toxicity. Instead, rate control may be achieved with beta-blockers, sotalol (Betapace), or digoxin (Lanoxin). Diltiazem (Cardizem, Tiazac, Tiamate) may be avoided because of its interaction with tacrolimus (Prograf) and cyclosporine (CsA, Neoral, Sandimmune, Gengraf), which interfere with metabolism, thus increasing drug levels and making it difficult to manage immunosuppression dosing in the early postoperative period.

Bleeding and Coagulopathy

Postoperative bleeding should be managed aggressively and coagulopathy identified and corrected. Ongoing bleeding with resultant transfusion requirements may compromise the lung transplant recipient because of aggressive volume loading, right ventricular strain, exposure to multiple donor antigens, and risk of further lung injury.

Renal, Electrolyte, and Fluid Balance

Renal function requires close monitoring during the early postoperative period because of aggressive efforts to maintain negative fluid balance and the concurrent titration of immunosuppression, antibiotic, antiviral, and antifungal agents that may impair renal function. Calcineurin inhibitors can be particularly nephrotoxic, and daily monitoring of drug levels as well as renal function and electrolyes is important for early identification of patients with worsening renal function to prevent potential toxicity.

Glycemic Control

Blood glucose levels may fluctuate early because of the intraoperative use of high-dose corticosteroids. Postoperative vasopressor use may also complicate glycemic management. The addition of chronic corticosteroids to the medical regimen after lung transplant may predispose patients to requiring chronic insulin.

INFECTION

Infection is a leading cause of mortality during the first year after lung transplantation and remains a major factor contributing to morbidity and mortality thereafter.[3,9,15] Infectious agents may be bacterial, fungal, viral, or from atypical bacterial or other opportunistic agents.

Vigilant surveillance for infection, rapid identification, and prompt directed treatment of infection is critical in the immunocompromised lung transplant population. Expanding criteria for recipient selection means that more patients with airway colonization with resistant bacteria may be considered for transplantation (cystic fibrosis and bronchiectasis). Patients are screened preoperatively, and positive sputum cultures are treated aggressively. In addition, at the time of transplant, swabs of the donor bronchi are taken in the operating room and sent for culture and sensitivity, and swabs of the recipient airways are sent as well. Attempts are also made to obtain, via the organ procurement agency, specific details of donor microbial culture and sensitivity reports from the referring hospital. Early postoperative antimicrobial management is then targeted to these specific organisms. All patients receive postoperative broad-spectrum prophylaxis against common Gram-positive and Gram-negative organisms (for eg, cefepime [Maxipime] for patients with no prior history of Methicillin-resistant *Staphylococcus aureus* [MRSA] colonization, or cefepime plus vancomycin [Vancocin, Vancoled] for patients with prior MRSA infection or colonization). Broad-spectrum prophylactic antibiotics may be continued until results from the intraoperative donor and recipient cultures are known. Culture-targeted antimicrobial therapy may then be continued for a period of 2 or more weeks, depending on the organism and its sensitivity pattern. Sensitive Gram-negative organisms may be treated for an 8-day course, whereas Staphylococcal infection or colonization may be treated for a full 2 weeks after transplant, because it may be more difficult to eradicate. In patients with highly resistant or multidrug resistant Gram-negative organisms identified preoperatively or in donor or operative cultures, the course of treatment may be extended even longer. In addition, patients with airway colonization or infection and ongoing air leaks from the pleural tubes may require an extended course of postoperative prophylaxis given the likelihood of colonizing the pleural spaces with the airway organisms, thus predisposing to possible development of empyema.

In addition to antibiotic prophylaxis, patients receive long-term prophylaxis against fungal and viral infections, as well as specifically against *Pneumocystis* infection.

Bacterial infection

Bacterial infection is common after lung transplant, with increased frequency within the first month and up to 1 year after transplant.[3] In addition, when patients are actively being treated for infection, immunosuppression must often be reduced to lower target levels, which may then increase the predisposition to subsequent development of rejection.

Both Gram-positive and Gram-negative organisms may be implicated in infection during the early postoperative period.[38] Pneumonia is common in lung transplant recipients and is treated with culture-targeted antibiotics. Of note, bacteremia in lung transplant recipients continues to be a problem, with one study reporting an incidence rate of 11.5% in a 2-center study.[39] The infections were both Gram positive and Gram negative, and the most common source of resistant Gram-negative bacteremia was pulmonary infection, with an overall mortality rate of 25% in the patients with documented bacteremia.[39]

Viral infection

Viral infections after lung transplant usually occur within the first 3 months postoperatively.[40] Opportunistic viral infections such as cytomegalovirus (CMV), Epstein-Barr virus (EBV), and other herpesviruses can be particularly problematic because latent virus can reactivate in patients previously exposed in the setting of immunosuppression therapy. Additionally, in previously unexposed recipients (seronegative recipients), virus can actually be transmitted via the solid organ transplant and patients may present with new onset of CMV, EBV, or herpesvirus infections. Typically, screening is performed on all recipients before transplant as well as on donors. Recipients who are seronegative (no prior exposure) receiving organs from seropositive donors are at highest risk of developing primary infection, which can be severe and life-threatening in the setting of immunosuppression.[38] Therefore, all lung transplant recipients receive long-term prophylaxis against these common viral organisms, beginning immediately after surgery, and recipients who are mismatched to donors (ie, seronegative recipient of seropositive donor) may receive higher dose prophylaxis than patients previously exposed (ie, seropositive recipient with either seronegative or seropositive donor). Seronegative recipients with seronegative donors still receive prophylaxis because exposure to virus via transfusion or other environmental exposure can still predispose them to significant morbidity if CMV infection develops. Options for viral prophylaxis may include valacyclovir (Valtrex) or valganciclovir (Valcyte), or possibly CMV-immune globulin. Patients are routinely screened posttransplant (at our center, on a weekly basis) for evidence of CMV viremia with blood sampling for CMV. Manifestations of CMV infection can range from asymptomatic to severe, life-threatening disease.[40] Patients with evidence of reactivation of virus or new primary infection are treated aggressively with augmented dosing of oral valganciclovir, or intravenous treatment with ganciclovir (Cytovene), foscarnet (Foscavir), or cidofovir (Vistide) for resistant cases.[40] In addition, when patients receive augmented immunosuppression for treatment of a rejection episode, viral prophylaxis may be augmented as well for the next 2 to 4 weeks.

Other community respiratory viral pathogens can also cause significant morbidity in lung transplant patients. These include respiratory syncytial virus, influenza viruses, parainfluenza viruses, and adenoviruses, among others.[15,41] In lung transplant recipients, infection with these viruses may range from mild upper respiratory infections to severe life-threatening pneumonia.[41] Over the last several years, influenza and parainfluenza infection in lung transplant patients has been reported.[42,43] Lung transplant patients can experience significant morbidity with these viral infections, including, in one study, intubation and MV in 13% of 39 patients, and 1 death.[42] In addition, 64% of those patients showed some degree of concomitant lung rejection, indicating that these infections may have implications for the long-term function of lung allografts.[42,43] When patients are admitted with upper respiratory infection or fever with pulmonary infiltrates, bronchoalveolar lavage sampling should include testing for these community respiratory viral pathogens as well as for the common bacterial pathogens. Seasonal response may not be helpful because the majority of influenza cases in 1 series were reported during the winter months, but parainfluenza cases predominated during the summer months.[42]

Fungal infection

Like viral infection, fungal infection after lung transplant is associated with significant morbidity and, if invasive disease is present, significant mortality as well.[15] The most common organisms are *Candida* species and *Aspergillus*. Ischemia at the bronchial anastamosis may predispose to infection at these sites and can result in disruption of the anastamosis and invasive dissemination of disease.[15,44] In one study, fungal prophylaxis with voriconazole in lung transplant patients was noted to help to prevent invasive aspergillosis infections as compared with targeted therapy once *Aspergillus* was identified (treated with itraconazole with or without inhaled amphotericin (Fungilin, Abelcet, Fungizone).[45] However, a recent survey of active lung transplant program shows considerable variation among lung transplant centers in initiating antifungal prophylaxis, approach to prophylaxis (preemptive vs universal), and choice of prophylaxis agent or agents. A majority of centers surveyed reported using inhaled amphotericin alone or in combination with itraconazole (Sporanox).[46]

IMMUNOSUPPRESSION

Suppressing the immune system to prevent organ rejection remains a key component of all successful lung transplants. Balancing adequate immune suppression without placing the patient at risk for life-threatening infection or the development of subsequent malignancy is of prime importance. Calcineurin inhibitors (tacrolimus or cyclosporine) remain the mainstay of immunosuppression regimens. Adjunctive therapies usually include a purine synthesis antagonist (azathioprine [Imuran] or mycophenolate mofetil [MMF] [Cellcept]) and corticosteroids (methylprednisolone [Medrol]) or prednisone (Meticorten, Orasone, Deltasone).[47] **Table 2** outlines mechanisms of action for these and other agents used for induction, maintenance therapy, or rejection treatment in lung transplantation.

Maintenance Therapy

Immunosuppression regimens for lung transplant patients have continued to evolve since the first successful lung transplants were reported in 1986 using cyclosporine and azathioprine for immunosuppression.[47] According to the ISHLT Registry, there is no clear consensus on any one maintenance immunosuppression regimen.[3] Most centers use a combination of calcineurin inhibitor (cyclosporine or tacrolimus) plus a purine synthesis antagonist (azathioprine or MMF) in conjunction with corticosteroids for maintenance immunosuppression therapy. Tacrolimus is the most frequently used calcineurin inhibitor, and MMF is the most commonly used purine synthesis antagonist at 1 year after transplant, in patients also receiving corticosteroids (see **Fig. 2**).[3]

Table 2		
Classification and grading of pulmonary allograft rejection		
Grading	**Description**	**Histopathologic Findings**
Grade A	Acute rejection	Presence of perivascular and interstitial mononuclear infiltrates
Grade A0	None	
Grade A1	Minimal	
Grade A2	Mild	
Grade A3	Moderate	
Grade A4	Severe	
Grade B	Airway inflammation	Presence of small airways inflammation, lymphocytic bronchiolitis
Grade B0	None	
Grade B1R	Low grade	
Grade B2R	High grade	
Grade BX	Ungradeable	
Grade C	Chronic airway rejection	Obliterative bronchiolitis: presence of dense eosinophilic hyaline fibrosis
Grade C0	Absent	
Grade C1	Present	
Grade D	Chronic vascular rejection	Accelerated graft vascular sclerosis: presence of fibrointimal thickening of arteries and veins (applicable to open biopsy material but not transbronchial biopsy material).

Data from Stewart S, Fishbein MC, Snell GI, et al. Revision of the 1996 working formulation for the standardization of nomenclature in the diagnosis of lung rejection. J Heart Lung Transplant 2007;26:1229–42.

Lower acute rejection rates were reported with tacrolimus-based regimens compared with cyclosporine-based regimens, and the least rejection was reported in the tacrolimus plus MMF group.[3] In some patients, sirolimus (Rapamycin, Rapamune) is added to the maintenance immunosuppression regimen, and at 5 years posttransplant it was used in 16% of patients, most commonly in conjunction with a calcineurin inhibitor (see **Fig. 3**).[3]

Induction Therapy

In response to significant acute rejection episodes, particularly within the first posttransplant year and the significant impact of acute rejection on the later development of chronic rejection, interest in using induction therapy developed. Induction therapy involves administering an augmented dose of medication at the time of transplant or in the very early posttransplant period to aggressively suppress immune response. According to the ISHLT Registry, there is no clear consensus on the use of induction therapy or on the selection of induction agent(s). However, 62% of patients received induction therapy in the first half of 2008, so it appears that interest in using induction therapies is continuing to increase.[3]

The earliest agents used for induction therapy included polyclonal antibodies (antithymocyte globulin [ATG, ATGAM]) or monoclonal antibodies (muromonab-CD3,

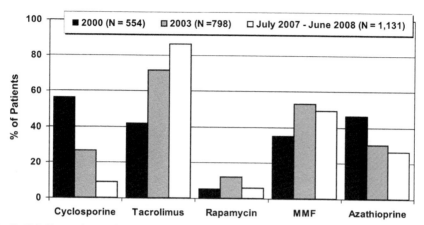

Fig. 2. This figure shows the maintenance immunosuppression being provided to adult lung recipients at the time of 1-year annual follow-up, as reported to the ISHLT Transplant Registry. Note the trends toward increasing use of tacrolimus and mycophenolate over the period between 2000 and 2008. Analysis is limited to patients receiving prednisone and alive at the time follow-up. Note: Different patients are analyzed in each timeframe. (With permission from The International Society of Heart & Lung Transplantation. Add J Heart Lung Transplant 2009;28:989–1049.)

OKT3 [Muromonab, Orthoclone]). Interleukin (IL)-2 receptor inhibitors are perhaps the most studied and, by the registry reports, the most commonly used induction agents. Daclizumab (Zenapax) is a humanized monoclonal antibody directed against the IL-2 receptor (CD25). After successful use in reducing rejection in renal and heart transplant recipients, it was studied in lung transplant recipients.[48] In comparison with historical controls without induction therapy and using the same baseline immuno-suppression regimen (tacrolimus plus azathioprine plus prednisone), daclizumab induction was found to decrease the incidence of grade 2 or greater acute rejection after lung transplantation without increase in adverse effects.[48] Subsequent to this, a prospective controlled trial comparing OKT3, ATG, and daclizumab-induction thera-pies for lung transplant concluded that there was no difference in development of acute rejection between groups, and less risk of infection in daclizumab patients compared with ATG and OKT3 patients.[49] Daclizumab was compared with ATG for induction in 3 studies with mixed results. ATG induction was found to be superior to daclizumab in reducing incidence and severity of acute rejection in one study,[50] whereas in two additional studies, daclizumab was found to be superior to ATG in reducing acute rejection.[51,52]

Basiliximab (Simulect), another IL-2 receptor antagonist, has been studied, also with mixed results. Basiliximab induction was compared with ATG induction and found to be inferior to ATG in reducing acute rejection and BOS in a single center report of 157 patients.[53] In contrast, basiliximab induction compared with historical control without induction was found to be superior in reducing rates of acute and chronic rejection, without increasing infection, and patients who were administered basiliximab had improved 2-year survival compared with control patients.[54]

More recently, induction therapy with alemtuzumab (Campath) has been reported in lung transplant patients. Alemtuzumab, a humanized anti-CD52 lymphocytic monoclonal antibody is administered just before transplantation. A single dose results in profound lymphoid depletion that may persist for up to 1 year after administration.[55]

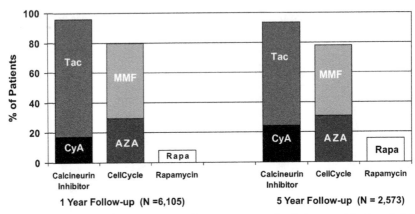

Fig. 3. This figure shows the maintenance immunosuppression being provided to adult lung recipients at the time of the 1-year and 5-year annual follow-up (January 2002 through June 2008) as reported to the ISHLT Transplant Registry. Note that the majority of patients receive tacrolimus and mycophenolate in both groups, and a general increase in the number of patients receiving rapamycin at the 5-year follow-up. Analysis is limited to patients receiving prednisone and who were alive at the time of follow-up. Note: Different patients are analyzed in year 1 and year 5. (To provide a snapshot of current practice, only follow-ups occurring between January 2002 and June 2008 were included. Therefore, this figure does not represent changes in practice between the 1-year follow-up and 5-year follow-up on a cohort of patients. The patients in the 1-year tabulation are not the same patients as in the 5-year tabulation). (With permission from The International Society of Heart & Lung Transplantation. Add J Heart Lung Transplant 2009;28:989–1049.)

Alemtuzumab induction was reported in 8% of lung transplant recipients in 2008 in the ISHLT Registry Report.[3] In comparing alemtuzumab versus ATG induction and reduced maintenance with tacrolimus monotherapy with historical controls (daclizumab induction, with tacrolimus plus azathioprine plus prednisone maintenance therapy), freedom from rejection was significantly greater with alemtuzumab than with either ATG or daclizumab induction.[56] Subsequent to this, alemtuzumab induction with reduced dose maintenance therapy (tacrolimus, lower-dose MMF and prednisone) compared with no induction therapy and standard maintenance triple drug therapy revealed comparable early survival rates, as well as rates of rejection and infection.[55] It appears that induction in theory is accepted as beneficial in reducing acute rejection, possibly impacting chronic rejection and possibly impacting survival. The optimal induction agent and maintenance immunosuppression regimen have still to be determined.

REJECTION
Acute Cellular Rejection

Organ rejection continues to be a significant limitation after lung transplantation, despite aggressive efforts to induce immune suppression and a multifaceted approach to immune suppression with respect to maintenance therapies. Acute cellular rejection (ACR) is common, with 36% of patients experiencing at least 1 episode in the first year,[3] and some reports estimating up to 90% of patients affected.[9,57] Most ACR episodes occur within the first postoperative year.[9] The presentation of acute cellular rejection can be quite variable and the true incidence is unclear because many episodes may be clinically unapparent, and only recognized if surveillance transbronchial biopsy has been obtained. Clinically, patients may be asymptomatic, or there may be nonspecific findings of increase in oxygen requirement, mild shortness of breath, or reduction in spirometry values; or clinically significant findings of fever, hypoxemia, and diffuse pulmonary infiltrates. Therefore, routine surveillance via bronchoscopy and transbronchial biopsy is done to identify the presence and severity of rejection episodes. Typically, the first biopsy is performed within the first 2 to 4 weeks, then at 3-month intervals thereafter for the first year. If rejection is identified and treated, interim repeat biopsies may be obtained to assess response to treatment, particularly in the absence of clinically significant findings. Frequency and severity of acute rejection are early indicators of developing serious rejection and are associated with the development of BOS, the clinical hallmark of chronic allograft rejection.[9,57,58]

Acute cellular rejection is graded according to the ISHLT grading system, revised in 2007. The grading system provides standard nomenclature and histopathological findings for each grade of rejection, and grades the amount of perivascular and interstitial mononuclear infiltrate (A grade), amount of small airways inflammation (B grade), presence of chronic airway rejection (C grade), and presence of chronic vascular rejection (D grade) (see **Table 3**).[59]

Treatment of acute cellular rejection

Treatment of acute cellular rejection depends on the severity of the rejection episode. Most mild and minimal (grades A1 and A2) rejection will not require specific treatment, unless persistent or clinically significant, or they may involve just raising the target levels of maintenance immunosuppression agents. Moderate and severe acute cellular rejection (grades A3 and A4) is usually treated first with pulse dose of corticosteroids (ie, 1 g of methylprednisolone daily for 3 consecutive days), or oral prednisone taper (100 mg/d, tapered to 10 mg/d over 14 days). Recurrent or refractory moderate and severe ACR may require additional treatment with any number of other therapies (additional pulse dose corticosteroid, IL-2 receptor antagonist, ATG, alemtuzumab). Additionally, baseline immunosuppression may be run at higher levels (for example, targeting higher tacrolimus levels, or increasing dosage of MMF).

Acute Antibody-Mediated Rejection (Hyperacute Rejection)

Acute antibody-mediated rejection of the lung is clinically associated with primary allograft failure and manifests very early after transplant. It typically occurs in recipients with preformed antibodies to donor human leukocyte antigens or endothelial cells.[59] Treatments may include plasmapheresis, intravenous immunoglobulin therapy, and augmented B-lymphocyte–targeted therapy (mycophenolate or azathioprine). Severe graft dysfunction may require extracorporeal membrane oxygenation support.

Chronic Rejection/BOS

Chronic rejection presents as BOS in lung transplant recipients. Patients with BOS experience progressive airflow obstruction postoperatively. Diagnosis is usually based on clinical findings, but surgical biopsy confirms the pathological lesion of bronchiolitis obliterans.[15] The development of BOS is usually a late complication and is the cause of death for most recipients surviving at least 1 year.[13] Although BOS does not present in the immediate postoperative period, patients diagnosed with BOS may require ICU management because of the declining lung function or

Table 3
Immunosuppressive agents used in lung transplantation, mechanism of action and clinical use

Class	Generic Name[a]	Mechanism of Action	Clinical Use
Calcineurin inhibitor	Cyclosporine	Suppresses IL-2 production by interfering with IL-2 gene transcription, thus inhibiting subsequent T-cell activation and T-cell–mediated immune responses[15,47]	M
	Tacrolimus	Suppresses IL-2 production by interfering with IL-2 gene transcription, thus inhibiting subsequent T-cell activation and T-cell–mediated immune responses[15,47]	M
mTOR kinase inhibitor	Sirolimus	Blocks IL-2–mediated T-cell activation[15,47]	I M R
Purine synthesis antagonist	Azathioprine	Antagonizes purine metabolism and inhibits DNA and RNA synthesis, thus inhibiting lymphocyte proliferation[15,47]	M
	Mycophenolate	Inhibits B- and T-lymphocyte proliferation by inhibiting nucleotide synthesis[15,47]	M
Corticosteroid	Methylprednisolone	Remove lymphocytes from the intravascular space and inhibit lymphokine-mediated amplification of macrophages and lymphocytes[15,47]	I M R
	Prednisone	Remove lymphocytes from the intravascular space and inhibit lymphokine-mediated amplification of macrophages and lymphocytes[15,47]	M R
Polyclonal antibody	Antithymocyte globulin	Reduces number and alters function of circulating T-lymphocytes[47]	I R
Monoclonal antibody	Alemtuzumab	Humanized anti-CD52 lymphocytic monoclonal antibody. Produces profound lymphocyte depletion by targeting CD52 antigen found on lymphocytes, monocytes, macrophages, and eosinophils[55]	I R
	Basiliximab	Chimeric (murine/human) monoclonal antibody. IL-2 receptor antagonist[47]	I
	Daclizumab[b]	Humanized monoclonal antibody. IL-2 receptor antagonist[47]	I
	Muromonab CD3[b]	Murine monoclonal antibody. Inhibits T-cell proliferation and differentiation[47]	I R

Abbreviations: I, induction; M, maintenance; R, rejection; mTOR, mammalian target of rapamycin.
[a] None are FDA labeled for use in lung transplant recipients.
[b] Daclizumab and Muromonab CD3 no longer manufactured.

the complications associated with increased immunosuppression. Numerous conditions are thought to be associated with BOS (ie, acute rejection episodes), but the cause(s) of BOS are not defined. Thus, there is no definitive treatment for the condition.[9]

SUMMARY

The ICU period is only one time point among many in the complex, multidisciplinary postoperative management required for patient survival and improved QOL. The care required on step-down units and after discharge to home each has unique care aspects that impact successful patient outcomes.

Research

Lung transplantation is evolving in all aspects based on research in the field. Although progress has been made in the last decade, standardized criteria for ideal recipient or donor selection do not exist. Postoperative management has been enhanced since the early period of lung transplants, yet there continues to be variability in practice across centers. Recipients of lung transplantation offer an unusual opportunity to study the impact of nervous system interruption of the vagus, sympathetic, recurrent laryngeal, superior laryngeal, and phrenic nerves on the regulation of ventilation, swallowing, and diaphragm and gastroesophageal functioning. Ongoing research in these areas may have implications for future advancements in patient care.

Currently, the main outcome criteria are survival and prolonged life for a patient with end-stage lung disease. There is discussion that QOL issues should be recognized as important an outcome as survival.[2] Studies have looked at health-related QOL issues in the lung transplant recipient.[60–63] These studies had sample sizes ranging from 10 to 304 patients. Other investigators have studied physical function outcomes with a variety of assessment strategies at various time points in the postoperative period.[64] In general, surviving patients report improvement if their condition is perceived as better than at the pretransplant period.

Research is necessary to address gaps in knowledge, because a large amount of current practice is not evidence-based. Targeted areas for research are numerous, but some include increasing the lung donor pool[6] and expanding the donor and candidate selection criteria. Other questions exist in regard to donor management, organ preservation and ischemic time, operative techniques, and preoperative and postoperative care strategies. Protocols to prevent and treat rejection and infection are significant areas for investigation. These numerous questions reflect the dynamic nature in the field of lung transplantation and characterize the ongoing inquiry and dedication of those providing care to lung transplant recipients.

Conclusion

The CCN with basic skills of ventilator management and hemodynamic assessment must add the components of immunosuppression, infection risk, and altered anatomy and physiology to care for lung transplant recipients. The knowledge and skill of the CCN to address the unique care requirements of the critically ill lung transplant recipient are essential in ensuring positive patient outcomes.

REFERENCES

1. Griffith BP, Bando K, Armitage JM, et al. Lung transplantation at the University of Pittsburgh. Clinical Transplant. Los Angeles: UCLA Tissue Typing Laboratory; 1992. p. 149–59.
2. McCurry KR, Shearon TH, Edwards LB, et al. Lung transplantation in the United States, 1998–2007. Am J Transplant 2009;9(4 Pt 2):942–58.
3. Christie JD, Edwards LB, Aurora P, et al. The Registry of the International Society for Heart and Lung Transplantation: Twenty-sixth Official Adult Lung and Heart-Lung Transplantation Report—2009. J Heart Lung Transplant 2009;28:1031–49.
4. Hardy JD, Webb WR, Dalton ML, et al. Lung homotransplantation in man. JAMA 1963;186:1065–74.
5. Orens JB, Estenne M, Arcasoy S, et al. International guidelines for the selection of lung transplant candidates: 2006 update—a consensus report from the Pulmonary Scientific Council of the International Society for Heart and Lung Transplantation. J Heart Lung Transplant 2006;25(7):745–55.
6. Van Raemdonck D, Neyrinck A, Verleden GM, et al. Lung donor selection and management. Proc Am Thor Soc 2009;6:28–38.
7. American Society for Transplant Physicians, Thoracic Society, European Respiratory Society, International Society for Heart and Lung Transplantation. International guidelines for the selection of lung transplant candidates. Am J Respir Crit Care Med 1998;158:335–9.
8. Kreider M, Kotloff RM. Selection of candidates for lung transplantation. Proc Am Thorac Soc 2009;6:20–7.
9. Orens, JB, Garrity ER. General overview of lung transplantation and review of organ allocation. Proc Am Thorac Soc 2009;6:13–9.
10. Mahidhara R, Bastani S, Rose DJ, et al. Lung transplantation in older patients? J Thorac Cardiovasc Surg 2008;135:412–20.
11. Baz MA, Palmer SM, Staples ED, et al. Lung transplantation after long-term mechanical ventilation: results and 1-year follow-up. Chest 2001;119:224–7.
12. Boujoukos A. Management of patents with heart-lung and lung transplants. In: Fink M, Abraham E, Vincent JL, et al, editors. Textbook of critical care. 5th edition. Philadelphia: Elsevier Saunders; 2005. p. 1969–74.
13. Trulock EP, Christie JD, Edwards LB, et al. Registry of the International Society for Heart and Lung Transplantation: twenty-fourth official adult lung and heart-lung transplant report—2007. J Heart Lung Transplant 2007;26:782–95.
14. Nathan SD. Lung transplantation: disease specific considerations for referral. Chest 2005;127:1006–16.
15. Lau CL, Patterson GA, Palmer SM, et al. Critical care aspects of lung transplantation. J Intensive Care Med 2004;19:83–104.
16. Orens JB, Boehler A, dePerrot M, et al. A review of lung transplant donor acceptability criteria. J Heart Lung Transplant 2003;22:1183–200.
17. Darby JM, Stein K, Grenvik A, et al. Approach to management of the heartbeating "brain dead" organ donor. JAMA 1989;261:2222–8.
18. Egan TM, Murray S, Bustami RT, et al. Development of the new lung allocation system in the United States. Am J Transplant 2006;6(5 Pt 2):1212–7.
19. Pochettino A, Bavaria JE. Anterior axillary muscle-sparing thoracotomy for lung transplantation. Am Thorac Surg 1997;64:1846–8.
20. Nador RG, Singer LG. Physiologic changes following lung transplantation. UpToDate 2010. Available at: http://www.uptodate.com/contents/physiologic-changes-following-lung-transplantation. Accessed June 18, 2011.

21. Veale D, Glasper PN, Gascoigne A, et al. Ciliary beat frequency in transplanted lungs. Thorax 1993;48:629–31.
22. Stanbrook MB, Kesten S. Bronchial hyperreactivty after lung transplantation predicts early bronchiolitis obliterans. Am J Respir Crit Care Med 1999;160:2034–9.
23. Trachiotis GD, Knight SR, Hann M, et al. Respiratory responses to CO2, rebreathing in lung transplants recipients. Ann Thorac Surg 1994; 58:1709–17.
24. Miyoshi S, Mochizuki Y, Nagai S, et al. Physiologic aspects in human lung transplantation. Ann Thorac Cardiovasc Surg 2005;11:73–9.
25. Starnes, VA, Lewiston NJ, Luikart H, et al. Current trends in lung transplantation. J Thorac Cardiovasc Surg 1992;104:1060–6.
26. Trulock EP. Lung transplantation. Am J Respir Crit Care Med 1997;155:789–818.
27. Boujoukos AJ, Martich GD, Vega JD, et al. Reperfusion injury in single-lung transplant recipients with pulmonary hypertension and emphysema. J Heart Lung Transplant 1997;16:439–48.
28. Norgaard MA, Andersen CB, Pettersson G. Airway epithelium of transplanted lungs with and without direct bronchial artery revascularization. Eur J Cardiothorac Surg 1999;15:37–44.
29. Siegelmann SS, Hagstrom JWC, Koerner SK, et al. Restoration of bronchial artery circulation after canine lung allograft transplantation. J Thorac Cardiovasc Surg 1977;73:792–5.
30. Couraud L, Bauded E, Nashef SAM, et al. Lung transplantation with bronchial revascularization. Eur J Cardiothorac Surg 1992;6:490–5.
31. Norgaard MA, Andersen CB, Pettersson G. Does bronchial artery revascularization influence results concerning bronchiolits obliterans syndrome and/or obliterative bronchiolitis after lung transplantation? Eur J Cardiothorac Surg 1998;14:311–8.
32. Maziak DE, Maurer JR, Kesten S. Diaphragmatic paralysis: a complication of lung transplantation. Ann Thorac Surg 1996;61:170–3.
33. Wanke T, Merkle M, Formanek D, et al. Effect of lung transplantation on diaphragmatic functioning patients with chronic obstructive lung disease. Thorax 1994;49: 459–64.
34. Atkins BZ, Trachtenberg MS, Prince-Petersen R, et al. Assessing oropharyngeal dysphagia after lung transplantation: altered swallowing mechanisms and increased morbidity. J Heart Lung Transplant 2007;26:1144–8.
35. D'Ovidio F, Mura M, Ridsdale R, et al. The effect of reflux and bile acid aspiration on the lung allograft and its surfactant and innate immunity molecules SP-A and SP-D. Am J Transplant 2006;6:1930–8.
36. Christie JD, Carby M, Bag R, et al. Report of the ISHLT Working Group on Primary Lung Graft Dysfunction part II: definition. A consensus statement of the International Society for Heart and Lung Transplantation. J Heart Lung Transplant 2005;24: 1454–9.
37. Dizon JM, Chen K, Bacchetta M, et al. A comparison of atrial arrhythmias after heart or double-lung transplantation at a single center: insights into the mechanism of post-operative atrial fibrillation. J Am Coll Cardiol 2009;54:2043–8.
38. Carlin BW, Lega M, Veynovich B, et al. Management of the patient undergoing lung transplantation: an intensive care perspective. Crit Care Nurs Q 2009;32:49–57.
39. Husain S, Chan KM, Palmer SM, et al. Bacteremia in lung transplant recipients in the current era. Am J Transplant 2006;6:3000–7.
40. Patel R, Paya, CV. Cytomegalovirus infection and disease in solid organ transplant recipients. In: Bowden RA, Ljungman P, Paya CV, editors. Transplant infections. Philadelphia: Lippincott-Raven; 1998. p. 229–44.

41. Whimbey EE, Englund JA. Community respiratory virus infections in transplant recipients. In: Bowden RA, Ljungman P, Paya CV, editors. Transplant infections. Philadelphia: Lippincott-Raven; 1998. p. 295–308.

42. Vilchez R, McCurry K, Dauber J, et al. Influenza and parainfluenza respiratory viral infection requiring admission in adult lung transplant recipients. Transplantation 2002;73:1075–8.

43. Vilchez RA, Dauber J, McCurry K, et al. Parainfluenza virus infection in adult lung transplant recipients: an emergent clinical syndrome with implications on allograft function. Am J Transplant 2003;3:116–20.

44. Tollemar JG. Fungal infections in solid organ transplant recipients. In: Bowden RA, Ljungman P, Paya CV, editors. Transplant infections. Philadelphia: Lippincott-Raven; 1998. p. 339–50.

45. Husain S, Paterson DL, Studer S, et al. Voriconazole prophylaxis in lung transplant recipients. Am J Transplant 2006;6:3008–16.

46. Husain S, Zaldonis D, Kusne S, et al. Variation in antifungal prophylaxis strategies in lung transplantation. Transpl Infect Dis 2006;8:213–8.

47. Taylor JL, Palmer SM. Critical care perspective on immunotherapy in lung transplantation. J Intensive Care Med 2006;21:327–44.

48. Garrity ER Jr, Villanueva J, Bhorade SM, et al. Low rate of acute lung allograft rejection after the use of daclizumab, an interleukin 2 receptor antibody. Transplantation 2001;71:773–7.

49. Brock MV, Borja MC, Ferber L, et al. Induction therapy in lung transplantation: a prospective, controlled clinical trial comparing OKT3, anti-thymocyte globulin, and daclizumab. J Heart Lung Transplant 2001;20:1282–90.

50. Burton CM, Andersen CB, Jensen AS, et al. The incidence of acute cellular rejection after lung transplantation: a comparative study of anti-thymocyte globulin and daclizumab. J Heart Lung Transplant 2006;25:638–47.

51. Lischke R, Simonek J, Davidova R, et al. Induction therapy in lung transplantation: initial single-center experience comparing daclizumab and antithymocyte globulin. Transplant Proc 2007;39:205–12.

52. Ailawadi G, Smith PW, Oka T, et al. Effects of induction immunosuppression regimen on acute rejection, bronchiolitis obliterans, and survival after lung transplantation. J Thorac Cardiovasc Surg 2008;135:594–602.

53. Hachem RR, Chakinala MM, Yusen RD, et al. A comparison of basiliximab and anti-thymocyte globulin as induction agents after lung transplantation. J Heart Lung Transplant 2005;24:1320–6.

54. Borro JM, De la Torre M, Miguelez C, et al. Comparative study of basiliximab treatment in lung transplantation. Transplant Proc 2005;37:3996–8.

55. van Loenhout KC, Groves SC, Galazka M, et al. Early outcomes using alemtuzumab induction in lung transplantation. Interact Cardiovasc Thorac Surg 2010;10:190–4.

56. McCurry KR, Iacono A, Zeevi A, et al. Early outcomes in human lung transplantation with thymoglobulin or Campath-1H for recipient pretreatment followed by posttransplant tacrolimus near-monotherapy. J Thorac Cardiovasc Surg 2005;130:528–37.

57. DeVito Dabbs A, Hoffman LA, Iacono AT, et al. Pattern and predictors of early rejection after lung transplantation. Am J Crit Care 2003;12:497–507.

58. Estenne M, Maurer JR, Boehler A, et al. Bronchiolitis obliterans syndrome 2001: an update of the diagnostic criteria. J Heart Lung Transplant 2002;21:297–310.

59. Stewart S, Fishbein MC, Snell GI, et al. Revision of the 1996 working formulation for the standardization of nomenclature in the diagnosis of lung rejection. J Heart Lung Transplant 2007;26:1229–42.

60. Smeritschnig B, Jaksch P, Kocher A, et al. Quality of life after lung transplantation: a cross-sectional study. J Heart Lung Transplant 2005;24:474–80.
61. Kugler C, Fischer S, Gottlieb J, et al. Symptom experience after lung transplantation: impact on quality of life and adherence. Clin Transplant 2007;1:590–6.
62. Lanuza DM, Lefaiver C, McCabe M, et al. Prospective study of functional status and quality of life before and after lung transplantation. Chest 2000;118:115–22.
63. DeVito Dabbs, A, Dew MA, Stilley CS, et al. Psychosocial vulnerability, physical symptoms and physical impairment after lung and heart-lung transplantation. J Heart Lung Transplant 2003;22:1268–75.
64. Grady KL, Lanuza DM. Physical functional outcomes after cardiothoracic transplantation. J Cardiovasc Nurs 2005;20:543–50.

Helping Hands: Caring for the Upper Extremity Transplant Patient

Darlene Lovasik, RN, MN, CCRN, CNRN[a],*, Daniel E. Foust, RN, BSN[a],
Joseph E. Losee, MD[b], W.P. Andrew Lee, MD[c],
Gerald Brandacher, MD[c], Vijay S. Gorantla, MD, PhD[b]

KEYWORDS
- Hand transplantation • Upper extremity transplantation
- Reconstructive transplantation
- Composite tissue transplantation • Nursing care

Reconstructive transplantation, or composite tissue allotransplantation (CTA), is the umbrella term for transplantations composed of multiple tissues including skin, muscle, tendon, nerve, blood vessels, lymph nodes, cartilage, bone, and vascularized bone marrow. Such multiplicity of tissues differentiates CTAs from solid organs and makes them immunologically complex grafts. Skin, in particular, is highly antigenic/immunogenic.[1,2] Clinical CTAs that have been performed include hand, face, trachea and larynx, tongue, bone and joints, abdominal wall, uterus, tendons, nerves, and penis.

HISTORY

Modern transplantation began with the pioneering research of the biologist Sir Peter Medawar and a plastic surgeon, Thomas Gibson, during World War II.[3–5] They treated pilots and soldiers with severe burns with skin grafts, and provided the first insights into the phenomenon of allograft rejection in the setting of skin transplantation. In 1954, the first successful living related kidney transplant between identical twins was performed by a plastic surgeon, Joseph A. Murray and his team including John Merrill, Hartwell Harrison, George Thorn, and Gustave Dammin.[2–5] Two of these innovators received the Nobel Prize in Medicine, Medawar in 1960 and Murray in 1990, for their groundbreaking work that changed the face of organ and tissue transplantation. Murray is the only plastic

The authors have nothing to disclose.

[a] UPMC Presbyterian, 200 Lothrop Street, University of Pittsburgh Medical Center, Pittsburgh, PA 15213, USA

[b] Division of Plastic and Reconstructive Surgery, University of Pittsburgh School of Medicine, Pittsburgh, PA 15261, USA

[c] Department of Plastic and Reconstructive Surgery, Johns Hopkins University School of Medicine, Baltimore, MD 21205, USA

* Corresponding author.

E-mail address: lovasikdj@upmc.edu

surgeon to receive the award.[5] Roberto Gilbert Elizalde performed the world's first hand transplant in 1964 in Guayaquil, Ecuador; however, the immunosuppressive regimen was limited to azathioprine and steroids, and the graft failed in 3 weeks.[1–8]

Following advancements in solid organ transplantation and immunosuppressive medication, Dr. Jean-Michel Dubernard and colleagues in Lyon, France, completed a unilateral hand transplant in 1998 on a 48-year-old man with a traumatic hand amputation. The recipient was noncompliant in following medical advice and anti-rejection medication therapy, and the limb was subsequently amputated 29 months after the original surgery.[1,2,9–13] This adverse event demonstrated the critical impor-tance of thorough psychosocial assessment as part of the pretransplant evaluation, and increased debate regarding the ethical issues surrounding non-lifesaving tissue transplantation. The first hand transplant in the United States was performed in 1999 at Louisville Jewish Hospital, University of Louisville, by Warren C. Breidenbach, MD and his team on a 37-year-old man who had a left hand (dominant) amputation in 1985 from a firecracker explosion. The recipient had an extensive pretransplant evaluation, including a thorough psychosocial and support assessment, and this graft remains viable 12 years after transplantation.[1,3,5,6,8–15] The Louisville team performed six more unilateral hand transplants and one bilateral hand transplant on male recipients between 2001 and 2011. One patient's transplanted hand was amputated after 275 days due to ischemic complications secondary to intimal hyperplasia.[10] Other reconstructive transplants such as hands, arms, face, larynx, and abdominal wall transplantation continued to be performed in several centers across Europe, China, the United States, and South America. The first partial face transplant was performed in Amiens, France in 2005 by Dubernard and colleagues on a 38-year-old woman with traumatic injuries after a dog attack. This is currently the longest surviving recipient of a facial transplant at 6 years after surgery.[10] Over the same period, 17 more facial transplants followed, including some full-face grafts with bone and vascularized marrow components.[1,3,5,10,11,16] The first partial face transplant in the United States took place at Cleveland Clinic in Cleveland, Ohio. Maria Siemionow, MD, PhD was the lead surgeon who performed the reconstruction transplant for a 45-year-old woman with traumatic injuries as a result of a gunshot to the face.[1,5,10,11,17]

The International Registry on Hand and Composite Tissue Transplantation (IRHCTT), founded in 2002, has collected detailed information on a voluntary basis from CTA centers around the world and annually publishes an analysis of data including functional recovery, patient and graft survival, adverse events, and complications. At this time, 30 unilateral and 21 bilateral hand recipients have been reported—a total of 72 hand, forearm, and arm grafts in more than 50 patients.[9] The median age was 32 years old; 94% of the recipients were male; the time since hand loss ranged from 2 months to 34 years; and in 46% of cases, the level of amputation was at wrist. Other reconstructive transplant procedures that have been reported now total 43 cases.[9] One patient, who underwent a simultaneous face and bilateral hand transplant, died 65 days after surgery. In the Western countries (Europe and the United States), three patients lost their transplanted grafts: one from a bacterial infection on day 45, another as a result of intimal hyperplasia on day 275, and the third at 29 months for complications related to noncompliance with medical and immunosuppressive ther-apy. In China, it is estimated that between 7 and 11 hand transplants were removed when patients were lost to follow-up, or through unreported episodes of acute rejection, or noncompliance with or inability to afford immunosuppressive therapy.[9,10] In the world experience, at least one episode of acute rejection occurred within the first year for 85% of the recipients, but all episodes were reversible when they were reported early by compliant patients and treated in a timely manner. It is important to note that acute rejection is easily observed in hand transplant patients because it can be diagnosed on visual inspection and through skin biopsy. This may explain the higher incidence of rejection in CTA over organ transplantation. There were no reported cases of graft-versus-host disease. All patients participated in intense posttransplant rehabilitation, including physical therapy, occupational therapy, and electrostimulation (the majority for 5 days a week for 1 year). In follow-up of at least 1 year, 100% of the recipients developed protective sensibility, 90% developed tactile sensibility, and 84% developed discriminative sensibility. Extrinsic muscle function, the ability to perform grip and pinch activities, began first, followed by the development of intrinsic muscle recovery between 9 to 15 months posttransplant. Sensory-motor recovery correlated to the level of amputation with hand grafts demonstrating higher function than forearm or arm grafts. There were no significant differences between left and right grafted hands. Most patients received triple immunosuppressive therapy of low-dose steroid, tacrolimus, and mycophenolate mofetil (MMF) initially, although regimens were adjusted to the side effects of the medications. Seventy-five percent of recipients reported improved quality of life, and many have returned to employable status.[9–11]

INDICATIONS

Trauma, bone or soft tissue malignancies, systemic diseases including sepsis related to overwhelming infection, vascular disease, or congenital birth defects may result in amputation of the hand and arm. The loss of the upper extremity has a profound psychosocial effect from both aesthetic and functional aspects as well as impacting the ability to work or resume regular work activities. Prosthetic devices assist with functional motor activities of daily living; however, none, even advanced myoelectric prostheses, are able to provide sensation, replicate the actions of a native hand, or provide the psychological benefit of appearing "whole."

Potential candidates for unilateral or bilateral hand transplants had amputations of one or both hands above the wrist or below the elbow, although several above-elbow transplants have been performed recently (functional outcome is yet to be reported). Selection (inclusion and exclusion) criteria vary between programs, but in general recipients are between 18 and 65 years old and in good health. Outcomes and graft function are superior for younger patients and recipients with an amputation below the elbow than for proximal amputations and older patients with comorbidities.[6] In distal grafts (wrist level amputations), nerve regeneration is accomplished faster and the intrinsic muscles innervate earlier resulting in superior overall functional outcomes.[18] Hand transplantation and other CTAs are performed to improve the quality of life; however, there are significant risks to the surgical procedure as well as the complications from immunosuppressive therapy. These risks have been previously assumed by organ transplant recipients with life-threatening diseases. The surgeon and transplant team must provide an informed consent consisting of information about the available treatment options, possible complications of the procedure, patient responsibilities, and a realistic expectation for functional outcome of the transplanted hand. "The decision to undergo such an extensive and complex procedure in an attempt to improve one's quality of life while maintaining a complete understanding and acceptance of the negative impact that immunosuppressive therapy may have on overall health can only be made by a capable and competent adult."[6(p3)] Contraindications include sepsis, human immunodeficiency virus (HIV), active cytomegalovirus (CMV), Epstein-Barr virus, active tuberculosis, viral hepatitis B or C, malignancy, current intravenous (IV) drug use, systemic or limb-related neuropathies, or a tattoo on the donor transplant within the past 6 months.[6]

PATIENT EVALUATION

Patients who may be candidates to receive a hand transplant must undergo an extensive evaluation that begins with a series of screening tests. An extensive history and physical examination with standard serum laboratory panels are part of the initial evaluation, as well as infectious disease studies including hepatitis B and C, HIV, CMV, and herpes. Dual confirmation ABO-typing is done on initial evaluation. Antibody levels are checked regularly and immediately before the transplant for ABO antibodies. Tissue-typing for anti-HLA (human leukocyte antigen) antibody (HLA- A and B), panel reactive antibody studies, and crossmatching are obtained. The surgery may last more than 10 hours, so satisfactory respiratory and cardiac function is essential; pulmonary function tests and cardiology clearance, possibly including an echocardiogram, multiple gate acquisition (MUGA) scan or both, are also part of the evaluation. The bone, muscles, and vascular status of the affected limb or limbs must also be assessed through computerized tomography (CT) scan/angiography. The existing residual limb(s) may have changed since the amputation as a result of atrophy of the muscles and/or alterations in the tendons and vasculature, or reveal other signs of disuse.[6,18] Both skeletal and functional magnetic resonance imaging (MRI) are performed; skeletal MRI will provide critical information about the bony structure and soft tissue status while the functional MRI will provide baseline information on the function of the cerebral cortex in the region that controls the residual limb. Although this specific cortical area may not show activity in an amputee, experience with posttransplant testing in recipients has demonstrated increased cortical activity in the region that controls the new graft.[7,16,19] Dental consults are standard during the transplant evaluation because occult infections of the oral cavity can migrate quickly through the body of the posttransplant immunosuppressed patient. Hand therapists administer a battery of questionnaires, obtain specific measurements, and assess the functional status of the residual limb(s).

The psychosocial assessment of family support, social issues, and financial concerns is essential; it mirrors the evaluation for suitability for organ donation; however, an extensive psychological evaluation is also obtained. Issues including the impact of amputation, coping and adjustment with hand loss, history of prosthetic use and compliance, motivation for hand transplantation, emotional and cognitive preparedness, body image adaptation, level of realistic expectations, anticipated comfort with transplanted hand, personality organization/risk of regression, history of medication compliance/substance abuse, and social support system/family structure are reviewed and examined.[6,20] This assessment will ascertain the recipient's coping abilities, ability to self-regulate emotional distress, and ability to tolerate the expected stresses. It will also predict the ability to form a working relationship with the transplant team and compliance with follow-up.[6,20]

IDENTIFICATION OF DONOR

The regional Organ Procurement Organization (OPO) is responsible for identifying potential CTA donors, educating donor families, and obtaining consent for donation. If a potential donor is identified, the OPO coordinator will discuss CTA with the family/significant other(s). At this time in the United States, this is a separate consent process from organ donation. Testing will begin to match the donor and recipient on immunologic parameters. Blood group, limb dimensions, skin color and tone (complexion matched with a skin swatch), and gender (same sex preferred) are some of the characteristics matched along with evaluation of serologies for viral or bacterial infections. Clinical pictures and radiographs of the donor hand and arm are transmitted to the surgical team to enable a transplant decision. While the potential recipient

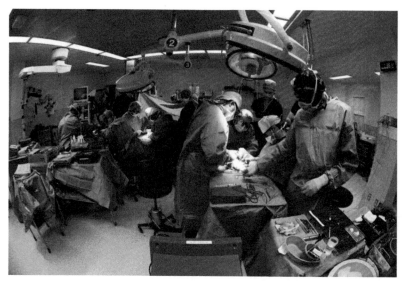

Fig. 1. Single hand transplant: UPMC surgical team led by W. P. Andrew Lee, MD. The donor team is preparing the graft in the foreground and the recipient team preparing the recipient in the background. (*Courtesy of* UPMC Medical Media Services.)

is traveling to the transplant center, the donor retrieval team is dispatched. The logistics and sequence of recovery vary, and limb retrieval may occur before or after organ procurement. The brachial vessels are cannulated and irrigated with a perfusion medium (HTK/Custodiol or University of Wisconsin solution) to wash out metabolites and sustain tissue viability during cold ischemia. The limb is packaged, stored in a cooler, and prepared for transport. The donor is fitted with a cosmetic matching prosthesis to allow for unaltered funeral practices.[6]

TRANSPLANTATION SURGERY

There is extensive preparation for the surgical procedure involving numerous members of the procurement, surgical, and transplant teams including: the logistics of setting up the operating room to accommodate up to four surgical teams (for a bilateral hand transplant), simulation of hand retrieval and hand transplantation, transportation workflow, transplant algorithm, and perioperative logistics. The OPO has detailed inclusion/exclusion criteria and all team members have the current waiting list with detailed recipient information. The transplant coordinator is key to synchronizing the sequence to transplantation, team mobilization and orchestration, and communicating clearly with all members of the team.[6,20]

The technical procedure for hand transplantation is fundamentally comparable to that for hand replantation. It is preferred that the donor and recipient limbs are prepared simultaneously on two different tables in the same operating room to facilitate communication between the two teams (**Fig. 1**). The preservation solution is flushed out of the donor limb, and excess skin and bone are removed. The radius and ulna are measured and the bones are shortened as necessary.[6,18] The arteries, veins, tendons, and nervous are identified, dissected, and tagged. The human hand has 27 bones, 28 muscles, 3 major nerves (radial, ulnar, medial), 2 major arteries (radial, ulnar), multiple tendons, veins, and soft tissue (**Fig. 2**). If the amputation resulted from explosives, meningococcal sepsis, or burns, the preparation of the stump

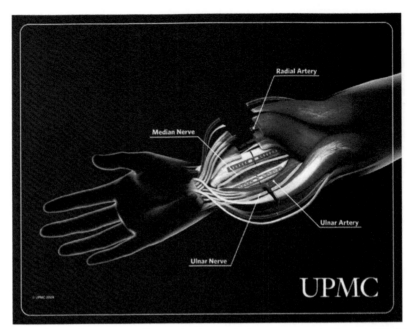

Fig. 2. Hand transplant surgery. Bones, tendons, arteries, nerves, and veins are attached by the surgical team in a surgery that can last as long as 11 hours. (*Courtesy of* UPMC Medical Media Services.)

must be performed carefully as the structures may be missing, avulsed, tenuous, atrophied, and/or encased in scar tissue.[6,18,21] The radius and ulna are cut to match the donor bones and internal fixation plates (low contact dynamic compression or T-plates) are used for osteosynthesis. The surgical sequence varies by team preference or needs of the operation. Sophisticated dual head operating microscopes are used to attach the arteries, veins, tendons (flexor and extensor—testing each tendon for function), and nerves (**Fig. 3**). The skin is closed with careful attention to flap positioning (Z plasty or 90–90 offset) to avoid circumferential pressure or scarring contracture and the hand and arm are positioned in a splint.[18] The flap is monitored by using both an implantable Doppler around one of the vessel anastomoses and two pulse oximeters, one on the finger of the transplanted hand and the second one on the control (either the contralateral, nontransplanted hand or the toes for bilateral hand transplants) (**Fig. 4**).[18]

THE PITTSBURGH EXPERIENCE

In an effort to limit the risks and side effects of multiple, high-dose immunosuppressant drugs that are required to prevent rejection, clinicians and researchers in reconstructive transplantation are exploring the successful strategies developed for organ transplantation. Utilizing research developed through the Thomas E. Starzl Transplant Institute at the University of Pittsburgh Medical Center (UPMC), the UPMC hand transplant team developed and implemented a new protocol based on the hypothesis that immunomodulation with donor bone marrow cell-based therapies would reduce long-term immunosuppression requirements. There are three components to the "Pittsburgh Protocol": induction therapy with alemtuzumab (30 mg),

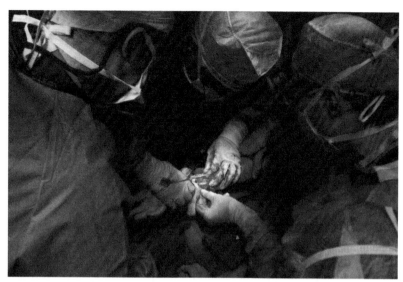

Fig. 3. Single hand transplant: UPMC surgical team led by W. P. Andrew Lee, MD. UPMC surgeons connect donor and recipient tissues during hand transplant surgery. (*Courtesy of* UPMC Medical Media Services.)

tacrolimus monotherapy (0.2 mg/kg/day) at 12 hours with an initial target trough of 10 to 12 ng/mL, and whole bone marrow cells (processed and cryopreserved from nine vertebral bodies of the respective donor) infused on day 14. At this time, five patients (three male and two female) have received this cell-based immunomodulatory protocol that reduces immunosuppression to low-dose monotherapy (**Table 1**). The protocol is efficacious and well tolerated, and episodes of acute rejection are low grade and infrequent. Functional, immunologic, and graft survival outcomes continue to be assessed during long-term follow-up.[6,22–25]

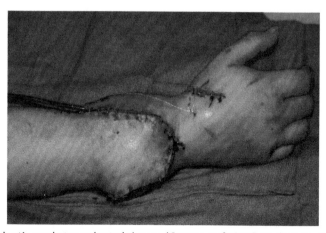

Fig. 4. Recipient's newly transplanted tissues. (*Courtesy of* UPMC Medical Media Services.)

Table 1
Patients who received upper extremity transplants at the University of Pittsburgh Medical Center (UPMC) 2009–2010

Patient	Amputation	Cause	Transplant Date	Graft
24-year-old man	Right hand	Military explosive	March 2009	Unilateral right distal forearm-level transplant
57-year-old man (First bilateral hand transplant in the United States)	Bilateral, mid-forearm	Strep A sepsis	May 2009	Bilateral mid-forearm transplant
41-year-old man	Bilateral, right above elbow and left distal forearm	Traumatic amputation—farming machinery	February 2010	Bilateral; right above-elbow arm and left wrist-level transplant
27-year-old woman	Right hand	Noro virus sepsis	September 2010	Unilateral right distal forearm-level transplant
33-year-old woman (First female bilateral hand transplant in the United States)	Bilateral, mid-forearms	Meningococcal sepsis	September 2010	Bilateral distal forearm-level transplant

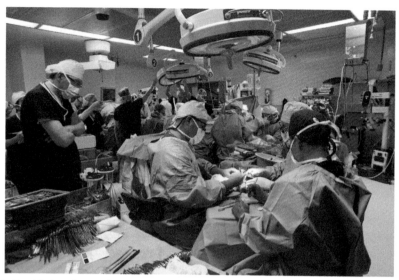

Fig. 5. Double hand transplant: UPMC surgical team led by W. P. Andrew Lee, MD. There are two donor surgical teams and two recipient surgical teams. (*Courtesy of* UPMC Medical Media Services.)

POSTOPERATIVE NURSING CARE
ICU Nursing Care

The patient is transported directly from the operating room to the intensive care unit (ICU) and a detailed report is provided to the ICU nurse. Standard ICU monitoring and (**Fig. 5**) patient care for the intubated postoperative patient and hemodynamic, circulatory, and fluid monitoring begins. Flap/replantation assessment includes capillary refill and pulse check every hour as well as hourly monitoring via the implanted Doppler and two pulse oximeters. In unilateral transplants, it is crucial to compare the waveforms and oxygen saturations between the new graft and the nontransplant contralateral control limb and alert the physicians if there is a change in status.[18] In bilateral transplants, this becomes a more challenging exercise and even subtle changes should be documented and reported. The transplanted limb is elevated in a Carter pillow, warm air blankets cover the limb, and the room is kept warm at 75°F (24°C) to prevent vasoconstriction. Pain management includes continuous nerve block(s) and IV narcotics as needed. The patient's fluid status, blood urea nitrogen (BUN), and creatinine are carefully monitored to assess the kidney function. The patient is at risk for acute tubular necrosis (ATN) due to a combination of events including the lengthy surgery, the release of endogenous nephrotoxins from muscles and tissues, and the initiation of immunosuppressive drugs. Dressings are changed by the surgeons, and hand therapists follow the dressing changes with a series of splints that are shaped to conform to the grafted arm. Tacrolimus dosing begins every 12 hours, and the tacrolimus target level is carefully monitored to maintain in the range of 10 to 12 ng/mL during the first several months.[22] Dosing is adjusted if the trough level is more than 20% below the target. Psychosocial support begins on arrival to the ICU because these patients **see** their transplanted hand(s); this is very different than the situation for organ transplant recipients. The ICU length of stay is determined by the individual patient's clinical status and outcomes.

Floor/unit Nursing Care

At UPMC, specific nurses were identified to provide continuity of care for the patients to ease the transition to the floor, and the nursing staffing was adjusted for a 1:1 patient ratio initially, then 1:2. The nursing staff continues to closely monitor the patients' vital signs and circulatory and fluid status. Capillary refill and pulse checks every hour and hourly monitoring via the implanted Doppler and two pulse oximeters are maintained as the nurses assess the grafted limb.[18] The continuous nerve blocks are usually discontinued in the ICU, and pain management is delivered via IV or oral narcotics. The nursing staff closely monitors the graft for signs of rejection; signs of rejection are clearly visible as maculopapular rash or scaling on the grafted limb.[6,23,26] It is equally important to monitor patients for infection because they have been immunosuppressed with the induction agents as well as the tacrolimus therapy.

As patients continue to improve, it is important to help them maintain control over their environment. The hand therapy sessions are scheduled for approximately 6 hours a day: a 3-hour therapy session in the morning, a 2-hour lunch and rest break, followed by a second 3-hour therapy session in the afternoon. The patients are active in their "Plan of Care," and we created an agenda for therapy and other activities so that the patients could anticipate and plan for their day. The nursing staff also provided extensive psychosocial support. One significant difference between the reconstructive transplant patients and the organ transplant patients is that these patients actually watch the progress of their transplanted organ. This may create anxiety when progress is slow or signs of rejection appear.

There were also some challenges that were not anticipated. The nursing staff looked forward to caring for this new patient population with both excitement and trepidation. The patients were functional within a range of activity with their prosthetic devices before surgery; however, they had significant physical care needs, including bathing, toileting, and eating after the surgery. Even small tasks such as changing the TV channel or scratching required assistance. The bilateral transplant patients used their legs to ring call light. During the postoperative period, caffeine is restricted and smoking is prohibited to prevent vasoconstriction of the blood vessels supplying the new graft.

Extensive patient/family education included teaching patients about their immunosuppressive medication, and the adjunct medications that are ordered including standard transplant prophylaxis such as sulfamethoxazole and trimethoprim (Bactrim) or inhaled pentamidine (aerosolized) to prevent *Pneumocystis* and other bacterial infections, and ganciclovir or valganciclovir for CMV prophylaxis. Skin and wound care is also essential. Specific safety instructions directed toward the loss of sensory protection are critical. Discharge planning is a team approach with the surgeons, nurses, hand therapists, social worker, patient, and caregivers. The patient remains in the region for several months to continue hand therapy while his or her transplanted limb continues to be carefully monitored during daily assessments in the outpatient transplant center.

Rehabilitation Therapy

Candidates for reconstructive transplantation receive a preoperative evaluation from the hand therapists, who continue to follow them closely through their postoperative course. After surgery, the patients receive a series of postoperative splints that are formed to the new graft(s). After the patient and graft are stable, patient care is directed to developing function with the newly transplanted limb. The progressive course of exercises is: protected passive range of motion (ROM), place and hold exercises, gentle finger and thumb flexion, forearm pronation/supination, forearm active ROM, and shoulder and elbow ROM. Therapy continues on an outpatient basis for several hours a day/5 days after discharge. The intensity and duration of therapy varies by level and laterality of transplant. The hand therapists play a vital role through positioning, splinting, therapeutic exercises, cortical reintegration, and training for activities of daily living to facilitate the independence of the upper extremity transplant patients.[27]

MONITORING FOR REJECTION

Signs of rejection are clearly visible on transplanted limb as a maculopapular rash, scaling, blistering, and edema. Skin and muscle biopsies are performed per institutional protocol to assess for evidence of acute rejection such as endpoint edema, erythema, and necrosis. The treatment for acute rejection includes the use of topical tacrolimus or clobetasol ointments as well as bolus steroids or antibody treatments as necessary. Chronic rejection manifests as intimal hyperplasia of the blood vessels of the graft structures including skin or muscle.[2,6,26] At this time, graft-versus-host disease has not occurred or been reported in CTA, including in those patients who have received whole donor bone marrow as part of their treatment regimen as part of the Pittsburgh Protocol.[2,3,7,9–11,22]

NERVE REGENERATION

Research has demonstrated that a major peripheral nerve that is rejoined microsurgically after complete severance may regenerate at a rate of up to 1 mm/day in adults. Long nerve homografts can also regenerate, but at a slower rate.[28]

Factors in successful peripheral nerve regeneration include surgical technical skills, nerve growth factors released by the recipients's own severed nerves, and the immunosuppression protocol chosen.[21] At this time, there is limited data on peripheral nerve regeneration in reconstructive transplantation. CTA is viable after revascularization, but not functional until the recipient nerves/axons regrow and replace the donor nerves to reinnervate the muscles and sensory end organs within the graft.[7] In rat model studies, tacrolimus appeared to contribute to peripheral nerve regeneration.[29] An increase in the speed of nerve regeneration was also described during clinical observations following CTA with tacrolimus immunosuppression.[28] At this time, prospective randomized human trials examining the efficacy of tacrolimus on peripheral nerve regeneration in CTA are pending.[21]

CORTICAL MAPPING

Recipients have functional MRIs performed to monitor the return of cortical function to the area of the brain that is responsible for controlling voluntary movement of the transplanted limb. This area of the brain has been dormant after the amputation, but testing reveals that function has resumed.[16,19]

FUTURE CHALLENGES

Debate continues among experts in reconstructive transplantation primarily focused on the risk/benefit balance. What amount of risk is too great for a non-life-threatening transplant? How does quality of life fit into the decision making? Should unilateral nondominant candidates be considered for surgery? Will nonadherence rates be similar to those for organ transplantation? The immunosuppressive therapy that is prescribed has multiple side effects that may cause potentially lethal complications including malignancy, infection, hypertension, nephrotoxicity, and metabolic disorders such as diabetes and renal failure. Most patients on immunosuppressive therapies also experience infectious complications. Graft failure due to infection or immunologic complications could lead to irreversible loss of function.[30–32] Broad acceptance of reconstructive transplantation as a safe and viable therapeutic option is dependent on reducing or eliminating the adverse consequences of immunosuppressive therapy. A 2009 survey of 474 surgeons/member of the American Society for Surgery of the Hand revealed diverse responses in their opinion of hand transplantation, with 34% in favor, 45% against, and 31% undecided. A majority of 69% considered the surgery high risk, although 71% considered it ethically appropriate when performed on a specific patient population. The loss of bilateral hands (78%) or the amputations of a dominant hand (32%) were the most accepted indications for hand transplantation.[33] This area will continue to be debated in both the public and medical literature; however, physicians and recipients believe that the results have been positive.

SUMMARY

Caring for upper extremity transplant recipients can offer challenges and opportunities to nursing staff in combining new patient procedures, new technologies, and complex patient care needs including unique physical care, monitoring and observation, rehabilitation expectations, and psychiatric/psychosocial support. Medical professionals continue to be apprehensive about the risks of immunosuppressive therapy and the possibility of acute and chronic rejection. The sustained development and research into reliable, reduced-dose immunosuppression or immunomodulatory strategies could expand the life-enhancing benefits of reconstructive transplantation.

REFERENCES

1. Swearingen B, Ravindra K, Xu H, et al. Science of composite tissue allotransplantation. Transplantation 2008;86(5):627–35.
2. Hautz T, Brandacher G, Zelger B, et al. Immunologic aspects and rejection in solid organ versus reconstructive transplantation. Transplant Proc 2010;42(9):3347–53.
3. Ravindra KV, Wu S, Bozulic L, et al. Composite tissue transplantation: a rapidly advancing field. Transplant Proc 2008;40(5):1237–48.
4. Shores JT, Brandacher G, Schneeberger S, et al. Composite tissue allotransplantation: hand transplantation and beyond. J Am Acad Orthop Surg 2010;18(3):127–31.
5. Tobin GR, Breidenbach WC 3rd, Ildstad ST, et al. The history of human composite tissue allotransplantation. Transplant Proc 2009;41(2):466–71.
6. Amirlak B, Gorantla VS, Gonzalez NR, et al. Hand transplantation. Available at: http://emedicine.medscape.com/article/1370502-overview Accessed August 20, 2010.
7. Brandacher G, Gorantla VS, Lee WP. Hand allotransplantation. Semin Plast Surg 2010;24(1):11–7.
8. Ravindra KV, Wu S, McKinney M, et al. Composite tissue allotransplantation: current challenges. Transplant Proc 2009;41(9):3519–28.
9. International Registry on Hand and Composite Tissue Transplantation. Available at: http://www.handregistry.com/page.asp?page=4. Accessed August 1, 2011.
10. Petruzzo P, Lanzetta M, Dubernard JM, et al. The International Registry on Hand and Composite Tissue Transplantation. Transplantation 2010;90(12):1590–4.
11. Petruzzo P, Lanzetta M, Dubernard JM, et al. The International Registry on Hand and Composite Tissue Transplantation. Transplantation 2008;86(4):487–92.
12. Lanzetta M, Petruzzo P, Dubernard JM, et al. Second report (1998–2006) of the International Registry of Hand and Composite Tissue Transplantation. Transpl Immunol 2007;18(1):1–6.
13. Lanzetta M, Petruzzo P, Margreiter R, et al. The International Registry on Hand and Composite Tissue Transplantation. Transplantation 2005;79(9):1210–4.

14. Breidenbach WC, Gonzales NR, Kaufman CL, et al. Outcomes of the first 2 American hand transplants at 8 and 6 years posttransplant. J Hand Surg Am 2008;33(7):1039–47.
15. Ravindra KV, Buell JF, Kaufman CL, et al. Hand transplantation in the United States: experience with 3 patients. Surgery 2008;144(4):638–43 [discussion 643-4].
16. Schneeberger S, Landin L, Jableki J, et al. ESOT CTA Working Group. Achievements and challenges in composite tissue allotransplantation. Transpl Int 2011;24(8):760–9.
17. Alam DS, Papay F, Djohan R, et al. The technical and anatomical aspects of the world's first near-total human face and maxilla transplant. Arch Facial Plast Surg 2009;11(6):369–77.
18. Azari, KK, Imbriglia JE, Goitz RJ, et al. Technical aspects of the recipient operation in hand transplantation. Transplant Proc 2009;41(2):472–5.
19. Frey SH, Bogdanov S, Smith JC, et al. Chronically deafferented sensory cortex recovers a grossly typical organization after allogenic hand transplantation. Curr Biol 2008;18(19):1530–4.
20. Amirlak B, Gonzalez R, Gorantla V, et al. Creating a hand transplant program. Clin Plast Surg 2007;34(2):279–89.
21. Jones NF, Schneeberger S. Arm transplantation: prospects and visions. Transplant Proc 2009;41(2):476–80.
22. Lee WPA, Gorantla VS, Schneeberger S, et al. A novel cell-based immunomodulatory protocol in hand transplantation—the Pittsburgh experience: level 4 evidence. J Hand Surg 2010;35(10):S51.
23. Schneeberger S, Gorantla VS, Hautz T, et al. Immunosuppression and rejection in human hand transplantation. Transplant Proc 2009;41(2):472–5.
24. Schneeberger S, Landin L, Kaufmann C, et al. Alemtuzumab: key for minimization of maintenance immunosuppression in reconstructive transplantation? Transplant Proc 2009;41(2):499–502.
25. Weissenbacher A, Boesmueller C, Brandacher G, et al. Alemtuzumab in solid organ transplantation and in composite tissue allotransplantation. Immunotherapy 2010;2(6):783–90.
26. Schneeberger S, Gorantla VS, van Riet RP, et al. Atypical acute rejection after hand transplantation. Am J Transplant 2008;8(3):688–96.
27. Pace J, Maguire K. Hand and upper extremity transplantation, a rehabilitation process. OT Practice 2011;16(8):17–22.
28. Owen ER, Dubernard JM, Lanzetta M, Kapila H, Martin X, Dawahra M, Hakim NS. Peripheral nerve regeneration in human hand transplantation. Transplant Proc 2001 Feb-Mar;33(1-2):1720–1.
29. Fansa H, Keilhoff G, Altmann S, Plogmeier K, Wolf G, Schneider W. The effect of the immunosuppressant FK 506 on peripheral nerve regeneration following nerve grafting. J Hand Surg Br 1999 Feb;24(1):38–42.
30. Bonatti H, Brandacher G, Margreiter R, et al. Infectious complications in three double hand recipients: experience from a single center. Transplant Proc 2009;41(2):517–20.
31. Brenner MJ, Tung TH, Jensen JN, et al. The spectrum of complications of immunosuppression: is the time right for hand transplantation? J Bone Joint Surg Am 2002;84-A(10):1861–70.
32. Wu S, Xu H, Ravindra K, Ildstad ST. Composite tissue allotransplantation: past, present and future-the history and expanding applications of CTA as a new frontier in transplantation. Transplant Proc 2009;41(2):463–5.
33. Mathes DW, Schlenker R, Ploplys E, et al. A survey of North American hand surgeons on their current attitudes toward hand transplantation. J Hand Surg Am 2009;34(5):808–14.

Transplant Infectious Disease: Implications for Critical Care Nurses

Sandra A. Cupples, PhD, RN*

KEYWORDS

- Transplant • Transplant candidates • Transplant recipients
- Organ donors • Ventricular assist devices • Infection
- Infectious disease • Critical care nursing

Solid organ transplantation increases both the length and quality of life for many patients with end-stage organ disease. However, transplantation is not without risk of serious complications, and infection is a major concern in this population. Critical care nurses are frequently involved in the clinical management of potential organ donors, transplant candidates with end-stage organ disease, and transplant recipients. The purpose of this article is to discuss infection in each of these patient populations, particularly with respect to the role of the critical care nurse in preventing, monitoring for, and treating infections.

BACKGROUND

There are several reasons why transplant-related infectious diseases are important to the critical care community. First, there are increasing numbers of immunocompromised patients in the intensive care unit (ICU) because of the improved survival rates of recipients of all types of solid organ transplants (SOTs). As the longevity of transplant recipients increases, these patients are more prone to develop chronic conditions that frequently require ICU stays. Second, the development of novel and more potent immunosuppressive agents has the potential to increase the frequency and severity of posttransplant infections that subsequently necessitate admission to a critical care unit. Lastly, infections in transplant candidates and recipients are a major cause of morbidity, mortality, increased length of hospital stay, and increased costs.[1]

INFECTIONS IN TRANSPLANT CANDIDATES

Transplant candidates are often at increased risk of developing infections due to their end-stage disease processes. These patients frequently require ICU care

Washington Hospital Center, 110 Irving Street NW, Washington, DC 20010, USA
* 9104 Wooden Bridge Road, Potomac, MD 20854.
E-mail address: sancupples@cs.com

Crit Care Nurs Clin N Am 23 (2011) 519–537
doi:10.1016/j.ccell.2011.08.001
0899-5885/11/$ – see front matter Published by Elsevier Inc.

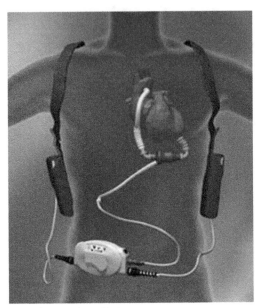

Fig. 1. HeartMate II VAD. (*Reprinted from* Thoratec Corporation; with permission.)

while they are on the transplant waiting list. Urinary tract infections are common in kidney and pancreas transplant candidates. Kidney transplant candidates are also at risk for infections in the native kidneys and occult abscesses. Liver transplant candidates may have intra-abdominal infections or aspiration pneumonia. Pneumonia is also common in the heart and lung candidate populations. Hospitalized candidates are at risk for catheter- or device-related infections, such as those associated with dialysis access devices or ventricular assist devices (VADs).

Patients With VADs

As of August 2011, there were more than 3100 candidates on the heart transplant waiting list in the United States.[2] To date, only 949 heart transplant procedures have been performed in the United States in 2011. Thus the demand for donor hearts far exceeds the supply.[3] VADs were developed to augment circulation in patients with end-stage heart disease. These devices have been approved by the Food and Drug Administration for three purposes: to bridge patients to heart transplantation, to bridge patients to recovery of their native myocardial function, and to provide permanent support for patients who are not deemed to be suitable heart transplant candidates ("life-time" or "destination" therapy).[4]

VADs can support the right or left ventricle or both. They stabilize the patient's condition by increasing cardiac output, improving perfusion to vital organs, and restoring mobility.[5,6] These devices are typically implanted through a median sternotomy incision and placed in a pre-peritoneal or intra-abdominal pocket.

The major components of a VAD are inflow and outflow cannulae, unidirectional valves, a polyurethane chamber (for pulsatile devices), and a pump or rotor. The device is connected to an external power source through a driveline that exits through the abdominal wall (**Fig. 1**).[7,8]

VADs contain biomaterials and, unfortunately, none of these materials are biologically inert.[9] Therefore, events that occur at the host–implant interface can trigger aberrant immune activation. When the patient's blood comes in contact with the foreign VAD surface, T cells can become activated and initiate a defective proliferative response and subsequent activation-induced cell death. As a result, the patient's immune system is impaired and the patient may be more susceptible to infection.[4,5,7,9]

Infection is a common complication of VAD therapy.[6] VAD-related infections may delay or prevent transplantation altogether and they are a major cause of morbidity and mortality in lifetime therapy patients.[10–12] The most recent International Society for Heart and Lung/Mechanical Circulatory Support Device Registry data indicate that infection occurred in 32.5% of the 655 VAD patients enrolled in this database and that patients with VAD infections had a 7.9% mortality rate.[13] Device-related infection rates reported in the literature have ranged between 13% and 80%.[5]

Potential infection sites include the surgical site or any component of the VAD (driveline, device pocket, or pump membrane). Driveline infections are the most common; however, more than half of all infections involve several device sites simultaneously.[7] VAD infections may remain localized or become systemic. If the infection spreads to multiple sites, serious complications such as bloodstream infections, bacteremia, sepsis, and endocarditis can ensue.[7]

Device-, patient-, and mechanical-related factors can contribute to VAD infections. Device-related factors include the exposure of percutaneous drivelines to pathogens and the VAD cavities and pockets that can harbor pathogens. These microorganisms can cause blood flow through the pump to become turbulent; this in turn enables the pathogens to adhere to the surface of the device.[4] Patient-related risk factors for infection include older age, poor nutritional status, indwelling catheters, prolonged intubation, postoperative bleeding, blood transfusions, multiorgan dysfunction, comorbidities such as diabetes mellitus and obesity, prolonged hospitalization before VAD implantation, and surgical reexploration.[4,6,7] Mechanical trauma to the driveline exit site is frequently associated with late-onset (>30 days after implantation) infections. Driveline trauma occurs when, for example, the controller or battery pack is dropped or when the driveline is snared on an object. These accidents result in shearing or torsion injuries that can lead to infection.[12]

Device-related infections can occur at any time; however, the majority develop between 2 weeks and 2 months of implantation.[7] Gram-positive pathogens, particularly *Staphylococcus* species, cause most infections.[14] These organisms are able to form a protective biofilm that blunts the host immune response and enables them to attach to and grow on inanimate surfaces.[8] Fungal and gram-negative bacilli, such as *Pseudomonas aeruginosa* and the *Enterobacter* and *Klebsiella* species, are other causative agents; these particular pathogens are associated with poorer outcomes.[4,7] The administration of broad-spectrum antibiotics often leads to the development of fungal infections.[7]

The clinical manifestations of VAD-related infections are varied. Presentation may be subtle or acute. If a device-related infection is suspected, the patient must have a thorough evaluation that includes a comprehensive physical examination and extensive work-up including blood cultures with Gram stains. If possible, cultures should be obtained before initiation of antimicrobial therapy.[7] Other sources of infection, such as pneumonia, urinary tract or catheter-related infections, must be investigated appropriately. Additional diagnostic tests are site specific. For example, ultrasound is used to evaluate suspected pump pocket infections; transesophageal echocardiograms are useful in the setting of VAD-related endocarditis. **Table 1** lists the typical signs and symptoms of device-related infections and potential treatment options.

The evidence regarding the impact of device-related infection and posttransplant outcomes is mixed. Some studies have indicated that these infections do not reduce 1-year[15] or overall[7,16] survival. Other studies have found that serious device-related infections can persist into the posttransplant period[7,17] and are associated with decreased early[11] and long-term[17] posttransplant survival. Although assist devices are often associated with infection, the benefits of this life-saving therapy are thought to outweigh the infection risk.[7] The major clinical implications for pre- and postoperative nursing care are listed in **Table 2**.

INFECTIONS IN POTENTIAL ORGAN DONORS

Infections can be transmitted via the allograft itself.[18] A donor-derived disease transmission is defined as "any disease present in the organ donor that is or has the potential to be transmitted to at least one of the recipients."[19(p234)] Donor-derived infectious diseases are rare. Unexpected transmissions, that is, those that were either unrecognized in the donor or for which the donor was not screened, occur in fewer than 1% of all solid organ transplantation procedures.[19] Although rare, these infections cause significant morbidity and mortality.

Factors that promote infection in potential organ donors include the use of medical devices and the treatment of patients in certain units that have high rates of bacterial contamination.[20] It is important to note that treatment of donor infections itself can further increase the potential donor's risk of iatrogenic infection, for example, via the insertion of intravascular catheters for antimicrobial therapy, the administration of immunomodulating medications such as corticosteroids, and prolonged hospitalization.[21]

Diagnosis of Infection In the Organ Donor

For a number of reasons, infections in potential organ donors may be difficult to diagnose:

- The donor may not have the clinical manifestations of infection due to insufficient numbers or virulence of pathogens.
- Hemorrhage or aggressive fluid resuscitation may dilute both organisms and serologic infection markers such that they are undetectable by conventional laboratory tests.
- The donor may not mount a fever response because brain death causes loss of temperature control and poikilothermia (a phenomenon whereby body temperature decreases to that of the environment).
- The donor's white blood cell count may be already elevated due to trauma, tissue inflammation, or medications such as corticosteroids.[21]

As a consequence, the diagnosis of infection may rely on culture and urinalysis reports, polymerase chain reaction (PCR) and nucleic acid testing results, characteristics of sputum, and changes in chest radiographs and computed tomography (CT) scans.[21]

Donor Screening

Potential organ donors undergo a rigorous infectious disease evaluation. Organ Procurement and Transplantation Network (OPTN) policies mandate that potential donors must be screened for the following pathogens: human immunodeficiency

Table 1
VAD infections: potential clinical manifestations and treatment options[4,7,8,34]

Infection Site	Potential Clinical Manifestations	Potential Treatment Options
Driveline	Poor wound healing Fever Leucocytosis Exit site abnormalities: • New or persistent serous drainage • Bleeding • Pain • Erythema • Necrosis Induration Nonintegration of driveline Wound dehiscence Simultaneous bloodstream infection	Wound care: • Débridement • Bactericidal agent Débridement and vacuum-assisted therapy Targeted systemic antimicrobial therapy Empiric therapy: gram-positive (especially staphylococcal) coverage
Pump pocket	New, persistent drainage from driveline exit site Manifestations of systemic illness: • Bloodstream infection • Fever • Leucocytosis Signs of local infection may or may not be present.	Targeted systemic antibiotics Empiric therapy: gram-negative coverage Débridement Open drainage Irrigation Relocation of driveline to clean exit site Implantation of antibiotic beads Replacement of device
Pump endocarditis (infection of any of the pump's surfaces)	Persistent fever Positive blood cultures Clinical manifestations of embolization to other organs (eg, brain, kidney) Progressive cachexia Mechanical problems: • Inlet obstruction • Outflow rupture • Bleeding or hematoma within device itself	Prolonged systemic antimicrobial therapy (4–6 weeks) Replacement of device

Table 2
Major clinical implications for preventing and treating VAD-related infections[4,6,14]

Preoperative	Postoperative
Removal of all unnecessary indwelling lines and catheters	Good handwashing techniques
Close monitoring and reporting of clinical manifestations of infection	Immobilization of the driveline at skin level (eg, with binder) per device manufacturer's recommendations
Maintenance of optimal blood glucose control	Strict sterile technique with cap and mask for dressing changes
Maintenance of adequate nutrition	Meticulous aseptic technique for driveline exit site care following device manufacturer's recommendations
Timely rotation of peripheral lines per protocol	Early extubation and ambulation
Maintenance of good oral hygiene	Removal of all invasive lines, drains, and catheters as soon as possible
Prompt administration of preoperative antibiotics	Prompt discontinuation of prophylactic antibiotics (typically 48 hours after VAD implantation)
Preoperative antiseptic prep per protocol	Close monitoring and reporting of risk factors for (eg, decreased albumin level; hyperglycemia, mechanical stress on wound/driveline) and clinical manifestations of infection
Preoperative clipping (not shaving) of surgical site	For patient with temperature above 38.3 degrees C: obtain and monitor white blood cell count and cultures (blood, sputum, urine)
Nasal culture; for *Staphylococcus aureus*, administer antibiotic ointment per protocol	Prompt administration of antimicrobial therapy as ordered Maintenance of adequate nutrition
	Maintenance of optimal blood glucose control Timely rotation of peripheral lines per protocol Maintenance of good oral hygiene

virus (HIV), hepatitis B virus (HBV), hepatitis C virus (HCV), syphilis, human T-lymphotropic virus (HTLV), cytomegalovirus (CMV), and Epstein–Barr virus (EBV). Blood and urine cultures are required for donors who have been hospitalized longer than 72 hours.[22] Potential heart donors are screened for toxoplasmosis. Many donors are also screened for nosocomial infections such as methicillin-resistant *Staphylcoccus aureus* or vancomycin-resistant enterocci. Because infection can be transmitted via transfusions, serologic testing is typically performed both before and after a potential donor receives blood products. In addition, family members are questioned about the potential donor's infection risk, including prior infection exposure, history, and immunizations; travel to endemic areas; and risky behaviors such as intravenous drug abuse. **Table 3** displays donor organ acceptance and exclusion criteria based on the results of infectious disease screening.

Table 3
Acceptance or exclusion of donor organs based on infectious disease testing[23]

Evidence of	Action
Active tuberculosis	Exclude from donation
Active systemic fungal infections	
Active rabies	
Active lymphocytic choriomeningitis	
West Nile virus or other encephalitis	
Antibody to human immunodeficiency virus	
Antibody to HTLV I/II	Generally exclude from donation except in life-threatening situations and with the recipient's informed consent
Hepatitis B surface antigen	Generally exclude from donation except in life-threatening situations, with recipient prophylaxis and with the recipient's informed consent
(Hepatitis B surface antigen positive or Hepatitis B core antibody IgM positive)	
Antibody to hepatitis C virus	Use only for recipient with antibody to HCV or for a severely ill recipient and with recipient's informed consent
Antibody to cytomegalovirus (CMV): base prophylaxis on recipient's CMV serostatus	Generally safe
Antibody to Epstein-Barr virus (EBV): Monitor EBV polymerase chain reaction if recipient is EBV seronegative	
Hepatitis B surface antibody (HBsAb) positive	
Rapid plasma reagin positive: Recipient should receive prophylaxis with penicillin	
Toxoplasma antibody positive: Seronegative heart transplant recipients should receive prophylaxis with trimethoprim/sulfamethoxazole (Bactrim; Septra); if recipient is allergic to sulfa, pyrimethamine (Daraprim) is used	

The acceptance of organs from donors with known infections with or exposure to HIV, hepatitis, or other viruses remains controversial.[21] Given that the number of transplant candidates on the waiting list far exceeds the number of available organs, strategies to expand the donor pool include accepting donors with certain infections, higher-risk serological profiles, and social histories suggestive of prior exposure to bloodborne infections as well as donors who may be more at risk for transmitting infections (eg, older donors and donors with long ICU stays).[20] Informed consent

---

Box 1
Principles of antibiotic selection and administration for potential organ donors[21]

1. Select a bactericidal antibiotic over a bacteriostatic antibiotic.

2. Use medication that will most directly target the identified bacteria to prevent the removal of harmless bacteria, the promotion of selective overgrowth of fungi, resistant organisms, or abnormal bacterial strains (eg, *Clostridium difficile*), and the development of gene mutations and highly resistant organisms.

3. Substitute directed antibiotic for broad-spectrum agent once sensitivities are available.

4. Follow Organ Procurement Organization antibiotic protocols for antibiotic selection.

5. Initiate empiric antibiotics when the potential risk of infection is high (eg, for open wounds, facial/sinus factures, pyuria) or in the setting of suspected bacterial infection (eg, suspicious chest radiograph findings; purulent sputum).

6. Base antibiotic selection on intensive care unit-specific tabulation of species and sensitivities (antibiograms).

7. Consider use of two antibiotics with different mechanisms of action to achieve additive synergy against gram-negative and gram-positive bacteria.

8. Consider empiric antibiotics for methicillin-resistant *Staphylococcus aureus* (MRSA) or vancomycin-resistant enterococci (VRE) in the ICU setting.

9. Consider antibiotics specifically effective against anaerobic bacteria in the setting of facial injuries, pulmonary aspiration, or contaminated wounds from an injury scene.

10. Administer antibiotics intravenously to maximize bioavailability.

11. Adjust antibiotic doses in the setting of renal failure, hepatic failure, and older donor age.

---

mandates that potential recipients be informed of the donor's infection status and the risk of infection transmission associated with that particular donor.[23]

Treatment of Infection In Potential Organ Donors

Effective treatment of bacterial infections in potential organ donors can result in successful transplantation.[21] **Box 1** displays important principles of antibiotic selection and administration for potential organ donors.

Role of the Organ Procurement Coordinator

The organ procurement organization's (OPO's) coordinator has major responsibilities regarding the prevention and treatment of infections and reporting known infections to transplant centers that could potentially receive organs from infected donors. Infections that must be reported to the transplant center are listed in **Box 2**. Moreover, all antimicrobial agents that are given to the potential donor must be documented and reported to each transplant center that receives an organ from that donor.[21]

Donor-Derived Disease Transmission

When a transplant center is informed that one of its organ recipients is confirmed positive for or has died from a potential donor-derived transmissible disease, that center must notify, within one working day, the OPO that procured that organ. The OPO must then notify the OPTN. These reports are forwarded to UNOS and uploaded to the Disease Transmission Advisory Committee's (DTAC's) secure website.

Box 2
Infections that must be reported to the transplant center[35]

Known conditions that may be transmitted by the donor organ must be communicated to the transplant center. These may include, but are not limited to, the following:

- Unknown infection of central nervous system (encephalitis, meningitis)
- Suspected encephalitis
- Hepatitis C
- Herpes simplex encephalitis or other encephalitis
- History of JC virus infection (causes progressive multifocal leukoencephalopathy)
- West Nile virus infection
- Cryptococcal infection of any site
- Rabies
- Creutzfeldt–Jacob disease
- Other fungal or viral encephalitis
- Bacterial meningitis
- Infection with human immunodeficiency virus (HIV) (serologic or molecular)
- Active viremia: herpes, acute EBV (mononucleosis)
- Serologic (with molecular confirmation) evidence of human T-lymphotropic virus (HTLV-I/II)
- Active hepatitis A or B
- Infection by *Trypanosoma cruzi, Leishmania, Strongyloides, Toxoplasma*
- Active tuberculosis
- Severe acute respiratory syndrome (SARS)
- Pneumonia
- Bacterial or fungal sepsis (eg, candidemia)
- Syphilis
- Multisystem organ failure due to overwhelming sepsis, such as gangrenous bowel
- Any new condition identified by the Centers for Disease Control and Prevention (CDC) as being a potentially communicable disease
- Any aspects of the donor's medical or social history that might increase the risk of disease transmission
- Donors at high risk for transmission of HIV

DTAC data indicate that, between 2005 and 2007, there were 80 donors with reported possible donor-derived infectious disease transmission, 30 recipients with confirmed (proven, probable, or possible) donor-derived infections, and 14 recipient deaths attributed to donor-derived infections. These deaths were due to hepatitis C, tuberculosis, HIV, Chagas disease, bacteremias, candidemia, *Strongyloides*, and lymphocytic choriomeningitis virus.[18]

INFECTIONS IN TRANSPLANT RECIPIENTS

There are three major factors that determine a transplant recipient's risk of infection. These include the patient's epidemiological exposure, either in the hospital or in the community; the patient's current antimicrobial regimen, if any; and the patient's net state of immunosuppression, which is defined as "the combined effect of all of the factors that determine the patient's susceptibility to infection."[24(p138), 25] The net state of immunosuppression includes the patient's current immunosuppressive regimen (number and strength of antirejection agents), as well as any of the following concurrent factors: infection with an immunomodulating virus (eg, CMV or EBV); metabolic or autoimmune disorders (eg, diabetes mellitus); neutropenia or lymphopenia; disruption of mucocutaneous barriers; and surgical sequelae (eg, fluid collections).[25]

Types of Infections

Approximately 80% of all transplant recipients have at least one significant infection during the first posttransplant year.[26] The three major groups of posttransplant pathogens are bacteria, viruses, and fungi (**Fig. 2**). Bacterial infections are the most common,[26] followed by viral and fungal infections.

Bacterial infections

Bacterial infections frequently occur at the transplant site. Bacterial pneumonias are common among all types of solid organ transplant recipients. Nosocomial pathogens of particular concern include *Clostridium difficile*, vancomycin-resistant enterococcus, methicillin-resistant *Staphylococcus aureus*, and extended-spectrum β-lactamase gram-negative bacilli. Common organ-specific bacterial infections and associated risk factors are listed in **Table 4**.

Viral infections

Most posttransplant viral infections are caused by two groups of pathogens: the herpes viruses (CMV, EBV, HSV 1 and 2, and varicella zoster) and the hepatitis viruses. Viral infections are particularly deleterious because they have both direct and indirect effects. The direct effect is the clinical syndrome caused by the virus itself, such as CMV pneumonia or hepatitis. Indirect effects include potential injury to the allograft, rejection, oncogenesis, and the virus's ability to alter the net state of immunosuppression, thereby increasing the patient's susceptibility to other opportunistic infections. The herpes viruses are characterized by latency. This means that once the virus is present, the patient will harbor the viral genome for life. Immunosuppression, particularly augmented immunotherapy in the setting of rejection, can trigger replication of latent herpes viruses.[24]

Cytomegalovirus is the most important pathogen that affects transplant recipients. There is a bidirectional relationship between CMV and rejection. CMV can trigger rejection and the inflammatory effects of rejection and rejection therapy can increase CMV viral replication. The allograft is more likely to be affected by a CMV infection than a native organ. Thus, liver transplant recipients with CMV infections are prone to develop vanishing bile duct syndrome, heart transplants recipients are at risk for coronary artery vasculopathy, lung transplant recipients are at risk for bronchiolitis obliterans, and so forth. The most common types of CMV disease are hepatitis, pneumonitis, and gastroenteritis. With regard to CMV serostatus, the risk of developing a posttransplant CMV infection is highest in CMV-seronegative recipients who receive an allograft from a CMV-seropositive donor and lowest in CMV-seronegative recipients who receive an allograft from a CMV-seronegative donor. Recipients who receive potent antirejection therapy such as antithymocyte globulin are also at increased risk for developing a CMV infection. A concurrent critical illness can lead to the reactivation of a latent CMV infection; this is thought to be associated with

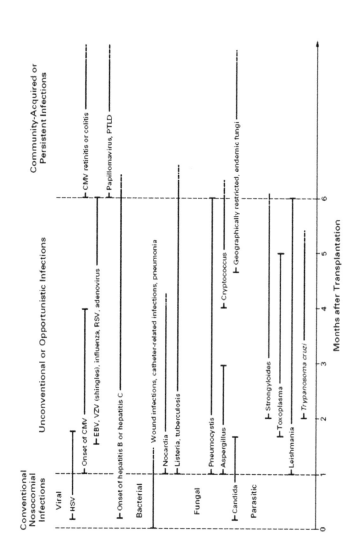

Fig. 2. Usual timeline of infections after organ transplantation. Exceptions to the usual sequence of infections after transplantation suggest the presence of unusual epidemiologic exposure or excessive immunosuppression. *Abbreviations:* CMV, cytomegalovirus; HSV, herpes simplex virus; PTLD, posttransplant lymphoproliferative disease; RSV, respiratory syncytial virus; VZV, varicella zoster virus. Zero indicates the time of transplantation. Solid lines indicate the most common period for the onset of infection. Dotted lines and arrows indicate periods of continued risk at reduced levels. (*Adapted from* Fishman A, Rubin RH. Medical progress: infection in organ transplant recipients. N Engl J Med 1998;338 (24): 1741-1751. Copyright© 1998. Massachusetts Medical Society; *with permission.*

Table 4
Organ-specific bacterial infections and risk factors

Type of Transplant	Common Types of Bacterial Infections	Risk Factors
Lung, Heart–lung[29,36]	Pneumonia Mediastinitis Sternal wound infection Anastomotic infections—may be secondary to placement of bronchial stents	Impaired cough reflex Poor mucociliary clearance Abnormal lymph drainage Disruption of phrenic nerve Prolonged mechanical ventilation Ischemia Reperfusion injury Bacterial colonization secondary to rejection-mediated airway inflammation Single-lung transplantation: infection in native lung
Liver[37,38]	Intra-abdominal (liver, biliary tract, peritoneal cavity) Surgical wound Cholangitis Abscesses Device-related Urinary tract Respiratory Bacteremia	Prolonged operative time; reoperation Blood transfusions Early rejection CMV infection Retransplantation Roux-en-Y choledocojejunostomy (due to reflux of intestinal material and microbial flora into the biliary system)
Kidney[24,29]	Urinary tract Surgical wound Infected lymphocele	Diabetes mellitus Renal insufficiency Prolonged urinary catheterization Neurogenic bladder Decreased urine flow Anatomic abnormalities Risk factors for recurrent urinary tract infections: • Serum creatinine >3 mg/dL • Prednisone dose >20 mg/day • Multiple treated rejection episodes • Chronic viral infections

(continued on next page)

Table 4
(continued)

Type of Transplant	Common Types of Bacterial Infections	Risk Factors
Heart[24]	Pneumonia Mediastinitis Sternal wound	Prolonged mechanical ventilation Prolonged intensive care unit stay Disruption of phrenic nerve Decreased pulmonary protective mechanisms Surgical reexploration Retransplantation
Pancreas, Kidney–pancreas[39,40]	Wound infection Intra-abdominal abscess Urinary tract infection Cystitis Peritonitis	Diabetes mellitus Kidney/pancreas transplant: anatomic reanastomosis of allograft Anatomic placement of organ: rate of deep wound infections higher with retroperitoneal placement than with intraperitoneal placement Prolonged urinary catheterization Neurogenic bladder Acidic pancreatic enzymes can cause anastomotic erosion and peritonitis Risk of cystitis higher with bladder drained pancreas due to effect of pancreatic enzymes
Intestine[30]	Device-related Pneumonia Translocation of bacteria from allograft to: • Peritoneal cavity • Portal circulation • Splanchnic venous system Bacterial overgrowth	Preoperative liver disease and/or sepsis Leakage associated with division of the lymphatics during procurement Preservation injury to intestinal epithelium Prolonged ischemic time; reperfusion injury Prolonged operative time; reoperation Inability to close abdominal wall Rejection High levels of immunosuppression Transplantation of intestinal contents and gastrointestinal flora with allograft Multiple invasive lines and catheters

proinflammatory cytokines and subsequent downregulation of the immune system. Agents used to prevent or treat CMV infection include ganciclovir, valganciclovir, acyclovir, and CMV immune globulin. Foscarnet is often used to treat ganciclovir-resistant organisms. Because CMV can be transmitted through blood transfusions, CMV-seronegative transplant candidates and recipients should receive CMV-negative, leukocyte-poor, or filtered blood products.[1,24]

Given that most adults are EBV-seropositive, most posttransplant EBV infections in adults are reactivated from latent pretransplant infections. However, EBV-seronegative recipients can acquire an EBV infection through blood transfusions or community exposure. The incidence of posttransplant EBV infections is highest in multiorgan and intestinal transplant recipients followed, in decreasing order, by kidney–pancreas, lung, heart, liver, and kidney recipients. Intravenous ganciclovir has been used as preemptive therapy for patients at high risk for EBV infections, for example, patients receiving antilymphocyte antibody therapy for rejection. The clinical sequelae of EBV infection range from a relatively mild mononucleosis-like syndrome to posttransplant lymphoproliferative disease (PTLD). Treatment options for mononucleosis include acyclovir. PTLD is a set of syndromes that ranges from a benign, self-limiting polyclonal proliferation of B cells to an aggressive, malignant, monoclonal lymphoma. Risk factors for PTLD include pretransplant EBV-negative serostatus, primary EBV infection, high EBV viral load, CMV serostatus mismatch (recipient is CMV negative and donor is CMV positive), CMV disease, potent rejection treatment, and type of allograft. The incidence of PTLD is highest in intestinal transplant recipients. Treatment options for PTLD range from antiviral agents (acyclovir, ganciclovir) and decreased immunosuppression for the benign polyclonal form to chemotherapy, radiation, resection, and decreased immunosuppression for malignant monoclonal lymphoma.

Fungal infections

Although invasive fungal infections have the lowest incidence of all infections, they are associated with the highest morbidity and mortality rates.[27] Risk factors for fungal infections include the use of high-dose corticosteroids and broad-spectrum antibiotics, rejection that requires increased immunosuppression, allograft dysfunction, and a simultaneous infection with an immunomodulating virus such as CMV.[24]

Two genera, *Aspergillus* and *Candida*, cause the vast majority of posttransplant fungal infections. Together, these two pathogens account for more than 80% of invasive fungal infections. These infections typically present during the first month posttransplant,[27] but they can occur at any time. The most common fungal infection that involves the respiratory tract is invasive aspergillosis, which may affect approximately 30% of solid organ transplant recipients.[28] Other portals of entry include the gastrointestinal tract and the skin. The risk of disseminated candidiasis is highest in neutropenic patients with central venous catheters who have received broad-spectrum antibiotics and who have had prolonged ICU stays.[29] Liver transplant recipients are at highest risk for invasive candidiasis, followed, in decreasing order, by pancreas, lung, heart–lung, kidney, and heart transplant recipients.[29]

INFECTIONS IN PEDIATRIC TRANSPLANT RECIPIENTS

Pediatric transplant recipients are often at higher risk for posttransplant infections for a number of reasons, including:

- Lack of immunity to common pathogens such as CMV and EBV
- Incomplete immunizations

- Increased technical difficulty and prolonged transplant operative time due to pretransplant palliative surgeries
- Inability to close the abdomen or chest due to placement of a large allograft into a small child
- Social behavior of children in densely populated day care and school settings.[30]

MEDIASTINITIS

Acute mediastinitis can develop after the implantation of mechanical circulatory assist devices or after heart, lung, and heart–lung transplantation. The risk of posttransplant mediastinitis is higher if the patient had a mechanical circulatory assist device or a total artificial heart as a bridge to transplantation. There are preoperative, intraoperative, and postoperative risk factors for mediastinitis. Examples of preoperative risk factors include diabetes mellitus, prior sternotomy, renal failure requiring dialysis, prolonged hospitalization before the transplant surgery, and obesity. The risk of developing mediastinitis is more than double in patients with a body mass index greater than 30. Intraoperative risk factors include blood transfusions and prolonged cardiopulmonary bypass, aortic cross-clamp, and operative times. Examples of postoperative risk factors include surgical reexploration, prolonged ICU stay, prolonged mechanical ventilation (>24–48 hours), having a tracheostomy, cardiopulmonary resuscitation, poor perioperative and postoperative glucose control, and low posttransplant cardiac output.[31]

The major etiologic pathogens associated with mediastinitis include, in decreasing order, gram-positive cocci (*Staphylococcus aureus, Staphylococcus epidermidis, Enterococcus* spp., *Streptococcus* spp.), gram-negative bacilli (*Escherichia coli, Enterobacter* spp., *Klebsiella* spp., *Proteus* spp., other Enterobacteriaceae, and *Pseudomonas* spp.), and fungi (*Candida albicans*).[31]

The initial clinical manifestations of mediastinitis may be subtle: mild chest pain, and edema or erythema along the sternal incision.[24] The most common presenting symptom is fever; it may be associated with localized infection, erythema, cellulitis, purulent drainage, pleuritic-like pain, and sternal instability. Diagnostic studies include CT scans, cultures, and laboratory tests. Laboratory findings include elevations in the white blood cell count, C reactive protein, and procalcitonin. The latter test is particularly useful in distinguishing between rejection and infection. Once mediastinitis is diagnosed, treatment should be initiated promptly. Therapeutic options include surgical drainage/débridement, wound irrigation, tailored parenteral antimicrobial agents, and nutritional support.[31]

NEUROLOGIC INFECTIONS

In transplant recipients, central nervous system (CNS) infections are among the most deleterious because they can be difficult to diagnose and treat. Diagnosis is often challenging because presenting symptoms, such as mental status changes, seizures, focal neurologic deficits, and headache, may be blunted by immunosuppressive therapy. Moreover, the neurotoxic effects of antibiotics, antiviral agents, and immunosuppressants themselves may make diagnosis even more complicated.[32,33]

The first step in diagnosing a suspected CNS infection is a neuroimaging study to establish the presence, location, potential etiology, and characteristics of any lesion(s). Magnetic resonance imaging studies of the brain or spinal cord or both are typically preferred to CT scans. Neuroimaging studies are useful in determining if the infection is focal or nonfocal and if it involves the meninges. Other diagnostic tests include cerebrospinal fluid analyses, electroencephalograms, viral polymerase chain reaction tests, cultures, and serologic tests. Brain biopsies are rarely done, except in the setting of posttransplant lymphoproliferative disease and brain abscesses. The posttransplant interval, patient-specific risk factors, and the timing and evolution of clinical manifestations also help to inform the diagnosis.[32]

CNS infections may be caused by fungi, viruses, or bacteria. Fungal infections carry the highest mortality rate—90% or higher—of all pathogens.[32] Most brain abscesses are associated with *Aspergillus.* These abscesses tend to occur early in the posttransplant period, particularly in recipients who have multiple risk factors for infection such as surgical reexploration, dependence on mechanical ventilation or dialysis, or retransplantation.[33] Unlike meningitis in immunocompetent patients, posttransplant meningitis is typically caused by fungi. In this setting, the patient often develops a systemic infection that subsequently spreads to the CNS. Viral CNS infections may be associated with the reactivation of a latent virus, such as JC virus-induced progressive multifocal leukoencephalopathy, or they may be caused by a new exposure to a pathogen such as West Nile virus. Other pathogens commonly associated with posttransplant encephalitis include the herpes simplex virus, varicella zoster virus, EBV, and CMV. Bacterial CNS infections are more frequently caused by *Listeria* and *Nocardia* rather than more common bacterial pathogens.[32]

Due to the severity of CNS infections in transplant recipients, an infectious disease consult, coupled with prompt diagnosis and treatment, is imperative. Empiric, broad-spectrum antimicrobial agents are typically administered until the causative organism is identified.[32]

FEVER

Immunosuppressive agents blunt the inflammatory response to infection; however, in most cases, transplant recipients with infections will have an increase in temperature. Some infections, however, tend to occur in the absence of fever. These include *Pneumocystis* pneumonia, focal fungal lung infections, and cryptococcal meningitis.[29]

Patients with a persistent fever greater than 38°C or acute pulmonary infiltrates or both are typically hospitalized for an infection workup. Fevers of unknown origin are most commonly associated with CMV or EBV viral syndromes. It is important to note that fevers in transplant recipients may also be caused by drug reactions (particularly antilymphocyte therapy), pulmonary emboli, deep vein thrombosis, and rejection. Rejection-induced fever typically occurs in lung transplant recipients. It occurs less commonly in kidney and liver transplant recipients and rarely in heart recipients.[24,29]

CARE OF TRANSPLANT DONORS, CANDIDATES, AND RECIPIENTS: IMPLICATIONS FOR CRITICAL CARE NURSES

Given that other human beings are the most frequent source of infection in the patient's environment, it is essential that nurses prevent the nosocomial transmission of respiratory viruses and the transmission of organisms through contaminated hands or inanimate objects.[29] In addition, it is important for critical care nurses to:

- Follow standard precautions
- Use aseptic techniques with vascular and urinary catheters
- Ensure that ventilator circuits, catheters, and dressings are changed per protocol
- Inspect all percutaneous catheter sites for signs of infection
- Maintain closed systems for urinary and suction catheters
- Keep the head of the bed elevated to decrease the risk of aspiration.

- Restrict access to patients by visitors and staff with colds or other contagious illnesses
- Avoid transporting transplant recipients through areas of hospital construction
- Promptly recognize and report the clinical manifestations of infections
- Obtain and report diagnostic test results in a timely manner
- Administer and document antimicrobial agents in a timely manner
- Assess and report the vaccination status of transplant candidates and recipients
- Know the CMV, EBV, and other pertinent serostatuses of the donor and recipient.[21,29]

SUMMARY

Infection is an important issue for critical care nurses as they care for patients throughout all phases of the transplant continuum: potential organ donors, transplant candidates, and transplant recipients. This article has reviewed salient issues relative to infections in each of these patient populations, including patients with VADs, and has highlighted key points pertaining to bacterial, viral, and fungal infections.

REFERENCES

1. Linden P. Approach to the immunocompromised host with infection in the intensive care unit. Infect Dis Clin N Am 2009 2009;23:535–56.
2. Organ Procurement and Transplantation Network. Waitlist overall by organ. Available at: http://optn.transplant.hrsa.gov. Accessed August 27, 2011.
3. Organ Procurement and Transplantation Network. Transplants by donor type. Available at: http://optn.transplant.hrsa.gov/latestData/rptData.asp. Accessed August 27, 2011.
4. Barnes K. Complications in patients with ventricular assist devices. Dimens Crit Care Nurs 2008;27(6):233–41.
5. Baddour L, Bettmann M, Bolger A, et al. Nonvalvular cardiovascular device-related infections. Circulation 2003;108:2015–31.
6. Richards N, Stabl M. Ventricular assist devices in the adult. Crit Care Nurs Q 2007;30(2):104–18.
7. Gordon R, Quagliarello B, Lowy F. Ventricular assist device-related infections. Lancet Infect Dis 2006;6:426–37.
8. Vinh D, Embil J. Device-related infections: a review. J Long Term Eff Med Implants 2005;15(5):467–88.
9. Itescu S, Schuster M, Burke E, et al. Immunobiologic consequences of assist devices. Cardiol Clin 2003;21:119–33.
10. Rose E, Gelijns A, Moskowitz A, et al. For the Randomized Evaluation of Mechanical Assistance for the Treatment of Congestive Heart Failure (REMATCH) Study Group. Long-term mechanical left ventricular assistance for end-stage heart failure. N Engl J Med 2001;345:1435–43.
11. Simon D, Fischer S, Grossman A, et al. Left ventricular assist device-related infection: treatment and outcome. Clin Infect Dis 2005;40:1108–15.
12. Zierer A, Melby S, Voeller R, et al. Late-onset driveline infections: the Achilles' heel of prolonged left ventricular assist device support. Ann Thorac Surg 2007;84:515–20.
13. Deng M, Edwards L, Hertz M, et al. Mechanical circulatory support device database of the International Society for Heart and Lung Transplantation: Third Annual Report – 2005. J Heart Lung Transplant 2005;24:1182–7.

14. Holman W, Rayburn B, McGriffin D, et al. Infection in ventricular assist devices: prevention and treatment. Ann Thorac Surg 2003;75:S48–S57.

15. Schulman A, Martens T, Russo M, et al. Effect of left ventricular assist device infection on post-transplant outcomes. J Heart Lung Transplant 2009;28(3):237–42.

16. Sinha P, Chen J, Flannery M. Infections during left ventricular assist device support do not affect posttransplant outcomes. Circulation 2000;102(Suppl 3):III194–9.

17. Poston R, Husain S, Sorce D, et al. LVAD bloodstream infections: therapeutic rationale for transplantation after LVAD infection. J Heart Lung Transplant 2003; 2003(22):914–21.

18. Ison M, Hager J, Blumberg E, et al. Donor-derived disease transmission events in the United States: Data reviewed by the OPTN/UNOS Disease Transmission Advisory Committee. Am J Transplant 2009;9:1929–35.

19. Ison M. The epidemiology and prevention of donor-derived infections. Adv Chron Kidney Dis 2009;16(4):234–41.

20. Len O, Gavalda M, Blanes M. Donor infection and transmission to recipient of a solid allograft. Am J Transplant 2008;8:2420–5.

21. Powner D, Allison T. Bacterial infection during adult donor care. Prog Transplant 2007;17:266–74.

22. Organ Procurement and Transplantation Network. Policy 2.2. Available at: http://optn.transplant.hrsa.gov/PoliciesandBylaws2. Accessed March 19, 2010.

23. Fischer S, Avery R. The AST Infection Disease Community of Practice. Screening of donor and recipient prior to organ transplantation. Am J Transplant 2009;9(Suppl 4):S7–S18.

24. Cupples S, Dumas-Hicks D, Burnapp L. Transplant complications: infectious diseases. In: Ohler L, Cupples S, editors. Core curriculum for transplant nurses. Philadelphia: Mosby/Elsevier; 2008. p. 135–98.

25. Fishman J, Rubin R. Infection in solid organ transplant recipients. N Engl J Med 1998;338:1741–51.

26. Kawecki D, Chmura A, Pacholczyk M, et al. Bacterial infections in the early period after liver transplantation: etiological agents and their susceptibility. Med Sci Monitor 2009;15(12):CR628–37.

27. Grossi P. Clinical aspects of invasive candidiasis in solid organ transplant recipients. Drugs 2009;69(Suppl 1):15–20.

28. Maertens J, Meersseman W, Van Bleyenbergh P. New therapies for fungal pneumonia. Curr Opin Infect Dis 2009;22:183–90.

29. Dummer J, Thomas L. Risk factors and approaches to infections in transplant recipients. In: Mandell GL, Bennett JE, Dolin R, editors. Mandell, Douglas and Bennett's principles and practice of infectious diseases, vol 2. 7th edition. Philadelphia: Churchill Livingstone/Elsevier; 2010. p. 3809–19.

30. Kosmach-Park B, De Angelis M. Intestine transplantation. In: Ohler L, Cupples S, editors. Core curriculum for transplant nurses. Philadelphia: Mosby/Elsevier; 2008. p. 455–511.

31. Van Schooneveld T, Rupp M. Mediastinitis. In: Mandell GL, Bennett JE, Dolin R, editors. Mandell, Douglas and Bennett's principles and practice of infectious diseases, vol 2. 7th edition. Philadelphia: Churchill Livingstone/Elsevier; 2010. p. 1173–82.

32. Zivkovic S, Abdel-Hamid H. Neurologic manifestations of transplant complications. Neurol Clin 2010;28:235–51.

33. Singh N, Husain S. Infections of the central nervous system in transplant recipients. Transpl Infect Dis 2000;2:101–11.

34. Garatti A, Giuseppe B, Russo C, et al. Drive-line exit site infection in a patient with axial flow pump support: successful management using vacuum-assisted therapy. J Heart Lung Transplant 2007;26(9):956–9.

35. Organ Procurement and Transplantation Network. Policy 4.1. Available at: http://optn.transplant.hrsa.gov/PoliciesandBylaws4. Accessed March 19, 2010.

36. White-Williams C, Kugler C, Widmar B. Lung and heart-lung transplantation. In: Ohler L, Cupples S, editors. Core curriculum for transplant nurses. Philadelphia: Mosby/Elsevier; 2008. p. 391–422.

37. Bufton S, Emmett K, Byerly AM. Liver transplantation. In: Ohler L, Cupples S, editors. Core curriculum for transplant nurses. Philadelphia: Mosby/Elsevier; 2008. p. 423–54.

38. Flynn B. Liver transplantation. In: Cupples S, Ohler L, editors. Transplantation nursing secrets. Philadelphia: Hanley & Belfus; 2003. p. 151–71.

39. Blakely MD, Lepley D, Achanzar T. Pancreas and kidney-pancreas transplantation. In: Ohler L, Cupples S, editors. Core curriculum for transplant nurses. Philadelphia: Mosby/Elsevier; 2008. p. 557–81.

40. Mize J. Pancreas and simultaneous pancreas-kidney transplantation. In: Cupples S, Ohler L, editors. Transplantation nursing secrets. Philadelphia: Hanley & Belfus; 2003. p. 143–9.

Index

Note: Page numbers of article titles are in **boldface** type.

Crit Care Nurs Clin N Am 23 (2011) 539–546
doi:10.1016/S0899-5885(11)00052-9
0899-5885/11/$ – see front matter © 2011 Elsevier Inc. All rights reserved.

Printed and bound by CPI Group (UK) Ltd, Croydon, CR0 4YY

03/10/2024

01040461-0014